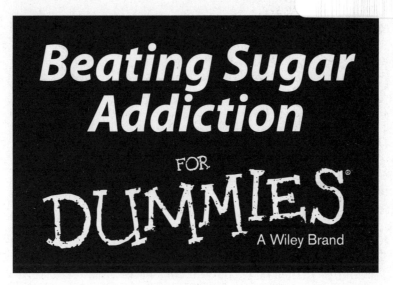

Beating Sugar Addiction

FOR DUMMIES®

A Wiley Brand

by Dan DeFigio

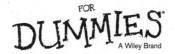

Beating Sugar Addiction For Dummies®

Published by
John Wiley & Sons, Inc.
111 River St.
Hoboken, NJ 07030-5774
www.wiley.com

Copyright © 2013 by John Wiley & Sons, Inc., Hoboken, New Jersey

Published by John Wiley & Sons, Inc., Hoboken, New Jersey

Published simultaneously in Canada

For general information on our other products and services, please contact our Customer Care Department within the U.S. at 877-762-2974, outside the U.S. at 317-572-3993, or fax 317-572-4002.

For technical support, please visit www.wiley.com/techsupport.

Wiley publishes in a variety of print and electronic formats and by print-on-demand. Some material included with standard print versions of this book may not be included in e-books or in print-on-demand. If this book refers to media such as a CD or DVD that is not included in the version you purchased, you may download this material at http://booksupport.wiley.com. For more information about Wiley products, visit www.wiley.com.

Library of Congress Control Number: 2013934758

ISBN 978-1-118-54645-1 (pbk); ISBN 978-1-118-54643-7 (ebk); ISBN 978-1-118-54649-9 (ebk); ISBN 978-1-118-54664-2 (ebk)

Manufactured in the United States of America

10 9 8 7 6 5 4 3 2 1

About the Author

Dan DeFigio is the owner and director of Basics and Beyond fitness & nutrition and works as a nutrition counselor, rehabilitative exercise specialist, and author in Nashville, Tennessee. Over his 20-year career, Dan has appeared on the *Dr. Phil Show* and in *SELF* magazine, *MD News,* and a slew of other media outlets. In addition to teaching exercise and nutrition, Dan is a former mixed martial arts fighter, and some say he is quite a piano player.

Dedication

This book is dedicated to the millions of people who struggle with achieving a healthy lifestyle — frustrated dieters, sugar addicts, diabetics, desk jockeys, frenzied soccer moms, and all those who can't seem to escape the whirlwind of stress and anxiety in their lives. May this book lead you toward empowerment, peace, and success.

This book is also dedicated to the wellness professionals who serve these millions — the doctors, nutritionists, therapists, fitness trainers, nurses, chiropractors, yoga teachers, and health coaches who lead the way for so many who desire to be healthier. If you've changed one life, you've made a difference.

Author's Acknowledgments

First and foremost, I want to thank the thousands of clients of Basics and Beyond fitness & nutrition (www.gettingfit.com) for your enthusiasm and dedication to wellness. Without your desire to improve yourselves, my team and I wouldn't have our fulfilling careers, and I wouldn't have had the experiences leading me to write this book.

In the "couldn't have done it without you" category, I'd like to extend special thanks to the staff at John Wiley & Sons, Inc. (www.wiley.com and www.dummies.com), especially Tracy Boggier for seeking me out for this project and Elizabeth Rea, Todd Lothery, Danielle Voirol, and Susan P. Watson for turning my nerdy ramblings into a readable *For Dummies* book.

I want to thank two giants in the nutrition science field: Dr. Michael Colgan (http://colganinstitute.com) and Dr. Thomas Incledon (www.human healthspecialists.com). The two of you are an inspiration to the nutrition science field, and we as nutrition professionals can't thank you enough for your enormous contributions to nutrition research and awareness.

Special thanks go out to Susan Carter B.P.E. at the Vanderbilt Center for Integrative Health (www.vcih.org) for your unbelievable passion and enthusiasm for this project. The world could use more people like you!

I owe a great deal to Dr. Mitch Johnson at the Center for Spiritual Living Nashville (www.cslnashville.org) and to Anke Nowicki (http://ankenowicki.com) for assisting my journey of self-inquiry and personal growth. Without the two of you, I couldn't be where I am today, and for that you have my eternal gratitude.

Publisher's Acknowledgments

We're proud of this book; please send us your comments at `http://dummies.custhelp.com`. For other comments, please contact our Customer Care Department within the U.S. at 877-762-2974, outside the U.S. at 317-572-3993, or fax 317-572-4002.

Some of the people who helped bring this book to market include the following:

Acquisitions, Editorial, and Vertical Websites

Project Editor: Elizabeth Rea

Acquisitions Editor: Tracy Boggier

Copy Editor: Todd Lothery

Assistant Editor: David Lutton

Editorial Program Coordinator: Joe Niesen

Technical Editor: Susan P. Watson, MS, RD, LD

Editorial Manager: Michelle Hacker

Editorial Assistant: Alexa Koschier

Art Coordinator: Alicia B. South

Recipe Tester: Emily Nolan

Nutritional Analyst: Angie Scheetz, RD

Cover Photos: Donut ©iStockphoto.com/ Turnervisual, Hammer ©iStockphoto.com/ ansonsaw

Composition Services

Project Coordinator: Sheree Montgomery

Layout and Graphics: Jennifer Creasey, Joyce Haughey

Proofreaders: Lindsay Amones, John Greenough, Judith Q. McMullen

Indexer: Rebecca R. Plunkett

Photographer: Shannon Fontaine (`http://shannonfontaine.com`)

Publishing and Editorial for Consumer Dummies

Kathleen Nebenhaus, Vice President and Executive Publisher

David Palmer, Associate Publisher

Kristin Ferguson-Wagstaffe, Product Development Director

Publishing for Technology Dummies

Andy Cummings, Vice President and Publisher

Composition Services

Debbie Stailey, Director of Composition Services

Contents at a Glance

Recipes at a Glance

Table of Contents

Introduction

* *

A high-sugar diet is one of the primary causes of obesity, diabetes, depression, stress and anxiety issues, and a host of other health problems. Sadly, a quick look at current healthcare statistics indicates that these "lifestyle" diseases are on a parallel rise across the board with the increase in sugar consumption.

I founded Basics and Beyond fitness & nutrition in 1993, and since then my team of experts and I have had the pleasure of changing the lives of thousands of people using exercise, stress management, and nutrition improvements. Over the last two decades, I've witnessed firsthand how rampant sugar abuse has become in the United States and how easily an otherwise smart and capable individual can become completely defeated by poor nutrition and a stressed-out lifestyle.

Sugar is just as addictive as cocaine, but it's cheap, legal, and socially acceptable. Sugar is pervasive too — consumption in the United States has increased fivefold in the 20 years I've been a nutrition counselor. Sugar addiction and other unhealthy lifestyle habits stem from (and result in) poor nutrition, lack of sleep, and stress. It's my hope that this book reaches many more people than I could possibly help in person and serves as a motivating guidebook and a beacon of hope for the millions of people struggling with sugar addiction, weight gain, stress, diabetes, and depression.

About This Book

Beating sugar addiction requires more than just staying away from sweet treats. To truly heal any addiction, you must look into the motivation behind your behavior, figure out what emotional holes you've been trying to fill with sugar, and understand how you've created a lifestyle that defaults to this unhealthy behavior.

I wrote this book with the intention of leading you through the process of getting off sugar and living a healthier lifestyle. As you go through the process, you'll find that it may also help you investigate, understand, and ultimately change your behavior and mind-set about lots of things — this is about much more than just cutting out sugar!

Herein you find chapters about understanding sugar, carbohydrates, and the psychology of sugar addiction; navigating restaurants and special occasions; eating mindfully; building a support system; revamping your kitchen; and — most important — breaking the cycle of failure and frustration, leading to a low-sugar life that's healthy, empowered, and under your own control.

Conventions Used in This Book

Throughout this book, I use the word *sugar* to mean a low-nutrient, sweet carbohydrate like table sugar, candy, sugared soda, or high-fructose corn syrup, as opposed to the technical definition of a sugar that a chemist would use. Other sources of carbohydrates you digest (like vegetables and grains) are technically broken down into simple sugars too, but I ask the chemistry geeks to forgive me as I use the word *sugar* in more conventional terms, referring to junk food and processed sweeteners.

Here are some conventions to keep in mind while digging into this book:

✔ I discuss a lot of health issues, but please understand that I refer to medical conditions and diseases in general terms only. You shouldn't consider the advice or information contained in this book to be pertinent to your specific situation — always consult with a qualified medical practitioner or nutrition consultant.

✔ I use *italics* for terms that I define or that I want to emphasize. Web addresses appear in monofont so they're easy to pick out.

✔ Part IV of this book is full of recipes, and in it I use the English system of measurement instead of metric, so temperatures are in Fahrenheit, measurements are in cups and ounces, and so on. The appendix provides information on metric conversions.

✔ In the recipes, do your best to use organic ingredients whenever possible. Eggs should be from pasture-fed, antibiotic-free chickens. Choose fresh fruits, vegetables, grains, and herbs that are organic to avoid pesticides and genetically modified ingredients. All meat will ideally be pasture-raised without hormones or antibiotics. Buy fish that is wild-caught, not farmed.

🍅 This tomato icon highlights the vegetarian recipes in the book.

What You're Not to Read

Some chapters contain *sidebars* — sections of text enclosed in boxes that give additional information, more technical details, or bonus advice that's not essential to the main text. If you're pressed for time, feel free to skip over the sidebars and perhaps come back to them later.

You can also jump over the items marked by the Technical Stuff icon. With these discussions, I go a little deeper into the science or technical details of a particular issue.

Foolish Assumptions

While working on this book, I made some general assumptions about who would be reading it:

- ✔ I assume that you feel stressed out and overwhelmed on a regular basis, and that you often resort to stress eating or medicating with sugar. And, most important, you want to stop doing this!

- ✔ I assume that you've struggled for a long time with losing weight, sticking to healthy eating plans, and getting control over your life in general, and you need dietary advice that's both effective and realistic.

- ✔ I assume that you have lots of things packed into your schedule, and you don't have all day to just sit around and read. I attempt to be reasonably thorough, without getting too technical or wordy, while delivering valuable information in a concise fashion. You can find additional information and resources online at www.BeatingSugarAddiction. com, including why diets don't work, simple ways to lose weight, how to do lunges without hurting your knees, and much more.

How This Book Is Organized

My (excellent) editors and I have divided this book into five parts to make the information more manageable and easier to take in. Each of the five parts of this book tackles a different aspect of beating sugar addiction. Here's how the information is organized.

Part 1: Are You a Sugar Addict or a Sweet Freak?

Part I delves into addiction, the long-term health ramifications of sugar abuse (the list may surprise you), and the science of sugar and why it's so addictive. In this part, you find out why some carbohydrates are worse than others, discover how to identify hidden sources of sugar, and understand why you should steer clear of artificial sweeteners. Another important objective of Part I is to help you uncover the emotional and psychological reasons that you may be abusing sugar, and to explain some of the common traits and behaviors of various types of sugar addicts.

Part II: Developing Your Low-Sugar or No-Sugar Food Plan

Part II is all about the things you need to know and do on a day-to-day basis to successfully wean yourself off sugar and start leading a healthier lifestyle. It starts with a basic overview of nutrition, portion control, insulin response, and nutrition supplements. You get crucial information about how nutrition affects your appetite and your sugar cravings, and I give you tips about how to adjust your daily eating to help you lose weight and stay off sugar.

Part II also walks you through the steps of overhauling your kitchen and pantry to aid your transition to a low-sugar household. The chapters get into shopping tips, deciphering labels, and figuring out what kind of food you should buy to keep yourself and your family healthy.

The last chapter of Part II delves into the benefits of detoxing from sugar and gives you suggestions for freeing yourself from other ugly addictions as well. I talk about finding a well-rounded doctor and give you some ideas about types of complementary medicine practitioners who may assist you in your quest to stay away from sugar and improve your health.

Part III: Living a Successful Sugar-Busting Lifestyle

In my opinion, Part III is the most important part of this book. This is where you find out what you need to do to identify triggers and avoid cravings. In fact, I lay out a step-by-step checklist that tells you exactly what to do when a craving strikes.

Eating mindfully (instead of reactively) is a huge part of successfully beating your sugar addiction, so Part III addresses mindfulness, willpower, and how to avoid becoming obsessive or neurotic about your diet.

In this part, I share some tips and techniques for eating out in a healthy, low-sugar fashion and also some ways for you to stay on track during the holiday season. One chapter in Part III shows you how to build a reliable support system for additional motivation and encouragement and prepares you for some of the reactions that you may not expect.

Lastly, Part III illustrates the importance of exercise and shows you how to set up a basic exercise system (complete with instructions and pictures) to lead you toward weight loss, more energy, elevated mood, and sugar-burning fun!

Part IV: Sugar-Busting Recipes

Part IV supplies you with 50 low-sugar recipes to kick off your new lifestyle. In addition to recipes for breakfasts, lunches, dinners, desserts, and snacks, you also find useful tips for staying prepared, understanding snacking success, bringing your family onboard, and upgrading your definition of dessert.

Part V: The Part of Tens

If you appreciate encapsulated lists of concepts and pointers, Part V is for you. Here you find out about ten foods that you may think are healthy but actually aren't. I've also assembled a list of the ten primary ways you can outwit your cravings — a short and to-the-point checklist of the most important principles of staying sugar-free.

Icons Used in This Book

Throughout the margins of this book you find symbols that spotlight important points, examples, and warnings. Look for these icons:

Tidbits and take-away messages are marked with this icon. These are nuggets that you may want to highlight or forward to your friends.

The Warning icon cautions you about something potentially harmful. When you see this icon, pay careful attention to the corresponding text.

This icon marks information that's important to remember, or it may represent a good summary of a larger section. These may be worth reading twice or jotting down if you're a note-taker.

Okay, I'll admit it — I'm a nerd. I love knowing the details of how and why things work the way they do, and nutrition science and physiology are not exceptions. Unfortunately for some of you, I also love to explain these details when I write. So if you're not into scientific explanations, feel free to skip the paragraphs marked with this icon. If you're a nerd like I am, enjoy the bonus information!

Where to Go from Here

You don't have to read *Beating Sugar Addiction For Dummies* from cover to cover before you begin your journey to free yourself from sugar! This book (like all *For Dummies* books) is written in modular fashion, with each chapter pretty much standing on its own. I hope that you read through each chapter eventually (because each one contains a lot of valuable information and food for thought that you may not already know), but you certainly don't have to read this book straight through.

Feel free to look over the table of contents, and peruse the section "How This Book Is Organized" earlier in this introduction so you can skip around to the topics that interest you most. In each chapter, I often direct you to other sections of the book that expand on a given subject or that give you more tips or information about the topic at hand.

For starters, I suggest that you read through Chapter 1 to get a quick overview of the major topics contained in this book — it's short, but it gives you a taste of everything so you can figure out what you want to read about next.

If you're ready to start making changes right away, move on to Chapter 2, where you can take the quizzes to find out which kind of sugar addict you might resemble and what some of your major motivations and mind-sets may be. After you understand the whys of your sugar problem, you can flip to Chapter 9 and start working on your sugar-free lifestyle right away!

If you'd like to find out more about sugar and how it affects your body (including why it's so addictive), spend some time on Chapters 3 and 4. If you feel like working out, Chapter 12 explains how to exercise for maximum results in minimal time.

Do you need help with making better food choices or doing a kitchen makeover? Chapters 5 and 6 are all about nutrition and how to overhaul your pantry, kitchen, and refrigerator. When it's time to cook, Part IV contains all the recipes for low-sugar breakfasts, lunches, dinners, snacks, and desserts.

If your theme has been, "I know what I'm supposed to do, but I'm just not doing it," flip to Chapter 8 to read about mindfulness and being intentional instead of reactive.

Whatever you choose to read first, enjoy it — and more important, implement it!

Part I

Are You a Sugar Addict or a Sweet Freak?

getting started with beating sugar

In this part . . .

✔ Take a quiz to determine what type of sugar addict you might be so that you can start understanding and changing your behaviors.

✔ Get to the physical, chemical, and emotional roots of why sugar is so addictive.

✔ Uncover the truth about carbohydrates and sugars — no, they're not all alike — and sort out good carbs from bad.

✔ Recognize some hidden sources of sugar and get facts about artificial sweeteners.

✔ Understand the effect sugar has on your brain as well as its negative effects on your overall health.

Chapter 1

Moving from Sugar Addiction to Sugar Reduction

. . . .

In This Chapter

▶ Explaining the nature of sugar addiction

▶ Taking the first steps of your low-sugar journey

▶ Turning your life around by changing your thinking

. . . .

*I*n small amounts, sugar is an innocuous substance. Every cell in your body needs sugar (glucose) to survive and function, so your digestive system breaks down the carbohydrates you eat into glucose to fuel your body. A major problem with the modern diet is that sugar is present in enormous amounts instead of in the small amounts found in natural foods. Processed foods, sweetened beverages, engineered sweeteners, and refined grains are pervasive in the Western food supply, overloading your body with unmanageable amounts of sugar and chemicals.

I'm not exaggerating when I say that sugar is just as addictive as cocaine. It acts on the pleasure center of the brain just like alcohol and heroin, so the more you eat, the more you want. Combine sugar's addictive nature with its omnipresence in society, and you get a recipe for a global health disaster. Reaching for yummy, quick, and convenient "food" during a stressful, time-crunched day is all too easy for people, and eventually they become addicted — both to the sugar and to the crazy lifestyle that leads them to it.

My goal is to guide you through the steps you need to take, both physically and emotionally, to wean yourself away from relying on sugar. This book will be helpful not only for the sugar addict but also for those who may not be truly addicted but who are searching for ways to decrease their reliance on stress eating and convenience foods in order to live a healthier lifestyle.

As you read this chapter, you'll start to understand the magnitude of the harmful effects that overdosing on sugar has on your body and the reasons why sugar can be so addictive. I share some easy tips to improve your eating without being neurotic or trying to be perfect. Best of all, you get a chance to start unraveling the psychology of your sugar abuse and to start looking at how you can begin to change your life by changing your thinking.

Understanding Sugar Addiction

As a species, humans evolved eating the small amounts of sugar found naturally in fruits and plants. Today, the modern American consumes more than 130 pounds of sugar each year, half of which comes from artificial corn sweeteners. Your body isn't designed to handle the massive load of sugar that the modern diet thrusts upon you, and the United States shoulders the embarrassing obesity, diabetes, and metabolic syndrome statistics to prove it, as shown in Figures 1-1 and 1-2. (Statistics compiled from the Harvard School of Public Health, the National Institutes of Health, and the Centers for Disease Control and Prevention.)

People are designed to crave high-energy foods like sugar. In nature, sweet taste means high calories, and to your ancestors, those calories could have made the difference between survival and starvation. Sugar also stimulates the release of feel-good chemicals in your brain, making you crave not only sugar's calories but also its sweet sensations.

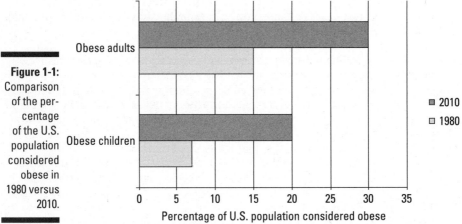

Figure 1-1: Comparison of the percentage of the U.S. population considered obese in 1980 versus 2010.

Illustration by Wiley, Composition Services Graphics

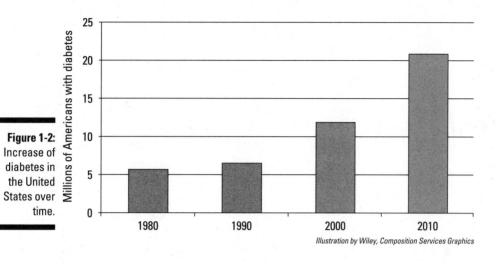

Illustration by Wiley, Composition Services Graphics

Figure 1-2: Increase of diabetes in the United States over time.

Defining sugar addiction

An *addiction* is anything that one must have to avoid a negative feeling or symptom, or the compulsion to artificially produce a pleasurable sensation. Sugar addicts use sugar as an energy booster (to avoid feeling tired and hungry) and a mood lifter because sugar triggers the production of *serotonin* and *dopamine,* which are hormones that make you feel happy and satisfied. (Alcohol and cocaine are other addictive substances that trigger serotonin and dopamine production.) As with drugs or other addictive substances, those who abuse sugar develop a tolerance to its effects and need more and more of it to yield the same rewards.

You're probably a sugar addict if one or more of the following descriptions rings true for you:

- ✔ Without sugar, you suffer extreme fatigue or have trouble concentrating.
- ✔ You eat sugar compulsively, even though you realize the negative consequences.
- ✔ You experience physical withdrawal symptoms if you go without sugar for a day or two.
- ✔ You find yourself obsessing over what your next sweet treat will be and when you get to have it.
- ✔ You hide your sugar consumption from other people or lie about your eating behavior.
- ✔ You need more and more sugar to experience the boost. Foods that used to taste sweet to you don't seem so sweet anymore.

> ✔ You repeatedly eat too much sugar, even though you promise yourself that you'll never do it again.
>
> ✔ You turn to sugar for an emotional lift, such as when you feel lonely or when you've had a bad day.

Weighing the global ramifications of sugar

Because overconsumption of sugar causes so many health problems, it places an enormous burden on an already struggling healthcare system (see Chapter 4 for more info on the health hazards of sugar and its consequences on the healthcare system). Here are some examples:

✔ **Shocking obesity statistics:** Obesity rates have doubled in the United States over the last 30 years, with a full two-thirds of Americans currently overweight or obese — making it statistically unusual not to be fat! The skyrocketing number of obese individuals worldwide runs parallel to the increase in the consumption of sugar and high-fructose corn syrup over the same 30-year span.

✔ **Diabetes woes:** The American Diabetes Association reports that about 9 percent of Americans, both children and adults, have diabetes, with millions more diagnosed every year. In addition, 80 million Americans have pre-diabetes (insulin resistance). The International Diabetes Federation estimates that global healthcare expenditures to treat diabetes and prevent complications total at least $465 billion annually.

✔ **Healthcare costs crisis:** The Centers for Disease Control and Prevention estimate that obesity costs the U.S. healthcare system more than $150 billion each year and that diabetic patients spend twice as much on healthcare as non-diabetic patients. With the consistent rise in the rates of obesity and diabetes in the developed world (along with the concomitant rise in related diseases and conditions), the cost of treating these "lifestyle diseases" will take a bigger and bigger chunk of your paycheck (see the following figure), until good nutrition and regular exercise become normal instead of health-nut behavior. (Statistics compiled from the Organisation for Economic Co-operation and Development, 2010.)

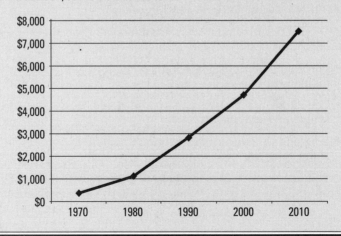

In Chapter 2, I categorize four types of stereotypical sugar addicts: the Exhausted Addict, the Sad Eater, the Undereater, and the Sugar Stalker. Head to Chapter 2 and take the quizzes to find out what kind of sugar addict (or which combination of addicts) you are so that you can figure out how best to change your eating habits and your lifestyle to become sugar-free.

Realizing how harmful sugar can be

Sugar, in all but the smallest amounts, is an addictive toxin and a driving force (or at least an aggravating factor) behind obesity, diabetes, liver disease, autoimmune disorders, chronic fatigue, hypothyroid disease, high cholesterol, osteoporosis, and metabolic syndrome.

These days the damaging diet begins in childhood, and as a result, young people are experiencing the devastating conditions and illnesses formerly reserved for the aging. Childhood obesity and diabetes are at an all-time high, leading most experts to believe that young people will have major problems much earlier in life because of their junk-food diet.

One of the most dangerous and seldom-discussed effects of a high-sugar diet is *tissue glycation*. Sugar causes a harmful chemical reaction in the tissues, forming molecules called *advanced glycation end products* (AGEs) that make your tissues stiffer and less elastic. The more sugar you eat, the more AGEs you develop, and these damaging molecules cause wrinkles, cataracts, stiff muscles, vascular disease, and brain damage — sugar literally shrinks your brain!

Getting Off Sugar without Driving Yourself Crazy

Despite what you may believe, getting off sugar and eating a healthier diet don't require superhuman discipline, some infomercial's "secret" pills, or a lifetime dedicated to eating like a rabbit. Try these easy steps to begin your journey, and consult Chapter 9 for more details:

- ✔ **Keep sugar and junk food out of your house.** You can't eat what you don't have! Remove the obvious culprits like soda, candy, brownies, cake, and pastries; also get rid of fruit juice, white flour products, dried fruit, energy drinks, and anything with the word *syrup* in the first five ingredients. See Chapter 3 for more information about carbohydrates and hidden sources of sugar that you may not be aware of, and consult Chapter 6 for tips on how to do a successful kitchen makeover.

✔ **Eat enough during the day.** Eating a combination of protein and carbohydrates (preferably from vegetables) every few hours helps keep your blood sugar levels stable and prevents your appetite from getting out of control. When blood sugar levels drop too low, you become ravenously hungry, and you're more likely to grab whatever convenience food is handy. Not eating enough during the day is one of the primary causes of overeating at night, which contributes to weight gain and late-night cravings. Turn to Chapter 5 for a lesson in putting together healthy combinations of protein and carbs throughout the day.

✔ **Get enough sleep.** Lack of sleep, stress, and sugar cravings create a vicious circle of frustration and fatigue. Stress keeps you up at night, so during the day you walk around exhausted, which increases your desire to use sugar as a convenient pick-me-up. High sugar consumption creates an inflammatory response in your body that creates more physical stress. Reducing your dependence on sugar does much more than just help you sleep better; visit Chapter 7 to find out additional ways that a sugar detox can benefit you.

✔ **Stop eating fat-free.** You may still be conditioned from the 1990s to think that fat-free versions of foods are healthier than their natural counterparts, but there's much more to the equation than just counting fat grams. Manufacturers of fat-free foods typically add more sugar and artificial ingredients to make up for the missing fat, so you do your body a favor if you stick to natural foods instead of fat-free, processed products. An exception to this is whole milk — it's a good idea to choose a lower-fat version (skim or 1 percent) that contains less saturated fat.

✔ **When you go out to eat at restaurants or special events, don't go hungry.** Restaurants are notorious for serving up three times as much food as you need (topped with lots of high-calorie sauces) and for presenting a tantalizing dessert menu to boot. Special events like parties and receptions are often sugar fests, with nothing but junk food and alcohol as far as the eye can see. To help you make sensible choices while you're out, eat a handful of a protein or high-fiber snack (such as a few bites of leftover chicken, a handful of almonds, or half an apple) before you head out. Chapter 10 is all about surviving restaurants, special events, and holidays.

✔ **Get regular exercise.** Exercise has more health benefits than anything else on the planet, period. Regular exercise helps stave off sugar cravings, boosts your energy, and tones your muscles. Exercise is essential for diabetics because it improves insulin sensitivity. Investigate Chapter 12 for an overview of constructing a basic exercise program that works for you.

✔ **Learn to identify and manage triggers and cravings.** If you're like most sugar addicts, you've learned to reach for something sweet under certain circumstances, like when you feel stressed, lonely, hungry, or tired.

To successfully reduce your sugar intake, you need to recognize these external triggers and practice making more conscious (and sensible) decisions when they present themselves. Chapter 9 — the most important chapter in this book, in my opinion — helps you determine what you really want when a craving hits.

✔ **Don't give up when you fall off the wagon.** People often get discouraged when they have a bad eating day, week, or month. Keep in mind that success is a series of ongoing decisions, and it's never too late to start making better ones, no matter how many poor decisions you've made in a row so far. All you have to work with is what you choose to do *right now,* so don't beat yourself up about the fact that you've been less than perfect in the past. Check out Chapter 8 for an introduction to mindfulness and avoiding reactive behavior.

Eating Right and Creating a New Normal

The reason diets don't work is that they don't lay out a realistic, sustainable plan that you can use to replace how you've been feeding yourself. Eating right doesn't require completely eliminating any one type of food (even sugar!) or some "revolutionary" new system of nutrition that has just been uncovered by scientists from another planet and is now available to you for only five easy payments of $49.95.

Eating well and losing weight requires a series of small, ongoing decisions that replace what you used to do most of the time. Aristotle said, in a nutshell, that we are what we repeatedly do, and excellence is therefore not a trait but a habit.

When you change what you usually do — that is, what's normal for you (see Chapter 9) — you get different results. No temporary diet can create a new normal for you; you must create one yourself by making different decisions most of the time.

Simplifying the low-carb concept

Low-carb eating is all about controlling your insulin levels. *Insulin* is a hormone that causes your cells to take up the glucose (sugar) that goes into the blood when you digest carbohydrates. Eating too many carbohydrates (or the wrong kind of carbohydrates) forces your body to produce a lot of insulin. Chronically high insulin levels cause conditions like metabolic syndrome, diabetes, high cholesterol, and polycystic ovarian syndrome. High insulin levels also promote fat storage and limit fat burning for energy. The primary way to keep your insulin levels low is to control your carbohydrate intake, both the type you choose and the amount you eat. Check out Chapter 3 for an in-depth discussion on types of carbohydrates and insulin control.

Carbohydrates are all broken down in your digestive system into simple sugars, but that doesn't mean that all carbohydrates are bad. Carbohydrates that break down faster raise your blood sugar levels more than carbs with a slower breakdown and release, and when it comes to blood sugar, slower is better. High blood sugar levels trigger a large insulin release, which causes fat storage and over time can cause diabetes and serious tissue damage.

To determine the effect that a particular carbohydrate has on your blood sugar, you can look up its *glycemic load* (see Chapter 5) to see how much a serving of that kind of carbohydrate raises your blood sugar levels.

High-fiber carbohydrates (like vegetables) generally have a lower glycemic load and therefore raise your blood sugar levels less than sugar (like candy or soda) or starchy carbs (like bread or pasta). Choosing vegetables over sugar or grains is a good way to start controlling your blood sugar levels, and adding protein and fat to the mix drastically slows the rise of blood sugar from the carbs in that meal.

Improving your eating with five easy habits

Chapter 5 is all about putting together a healthy nutrition system for yourself. Here are some tips to get you started:

- ✔ Eating a high-protein breakfast stimulates your metabolism, stabilizes your blood sugar, and keeps your energy levels high throughout the morning. An all-carb continental breakfast promotes fat storage and puts you on the blood sugar roller coaster for the rest of the day. See Chapter 13 for energy-boosting breakfast ideas.

- ✔ Vegetables should make up the majority of your carbohydrate intake (see Chapter 5). Vegetables are low in calories and high in vitamins, minerals, fiber, and phytonutrients, so they make the ideal carbohydrate choice. Fruits are high in nutrients, but they also contain more sugar, so be judicious in your portions.

- ✔ Try to eat a protein source every time you eat. Protein is essential for rebuilding muscles and organs and for making immune system cells, hormones, enzymes, and a host of other necessary components of a healthy physiology. Eating protein with carbohydrates slows down the release of sugar into the bloodstream, so getting enough protein is important for blood sugar control too. Protein helps keep your appetite at bay longer than carbohydrates do.

✔ Drinking enough water is important to keep all your body's tissues healthy, including your brain. Being dehydrated decreases your mental and physical functions and triggers your hypothalamus to turn on the hunger and thirst centers in your brain, increasing appetite and cravings. A general guideline is to aim to drink a minimum of 64 ounces of water every day.

✔ Using the right nutrition supplements is a good way to ensure that you supply your body with optimum nutrition. Nutrition deficiencies can cause food cravings and contribute to a host of degenerative diseases like arthritis, heart disease, and cancer. Chapter 5 explains which nutrition supplements may be helpful under certain circumstances.

Change your thinking, change your life

Overcoming your sugar addiction requires different behaviors and new ways of thinking. You need to not only improve your nutrition plan but also train yourself to make proactive, conscious decisions instead of acting reactively to stress.

Learning to be mindful and intentional instead of being reactive is a crucial component of controlling your eating and managing the stress in your life. Your diet starts with your brain, not with your mouth, so go through Chapters 8 and 9 to begin changing your life by changing your thinking.

Figuring Out What You Really Need Instead of Sugar

If you're like most addicts, you use sugar to medicate yourself. Sugar is a substitute for something that's missing in your life. To stop the cravings and heal your addiction, you have to figure out what emotional "hole" you're trying to fill with sugar.

The next time you have a craving for something sweet, stop to figure out what it is that you really want — chances are it's not sugar. Here are some examples:

✔ If you have the urge to grab something sweet when you get stressed, what you probably want is to feel peaceful and in control of your life. Sugar can't give you that.

✔ If you're ravenous when you get home at night and are ready to grab whatever you can stuff yourself with the fastest, what your body really wants is nourishment. Sugar can't give you that.

✔ When you desire sugar because you feel lonely, sad, or hopeless, what you probably want is companionship, hope, and joy. Sugar can't give you that.

After you start to recognize what your real motivations are, you can start taking steps to achieve those states instead of drugging yourself with sugar. Chapter 9 takes you through the process in more detail.

Chapter 2

Figuring Out Why You're Addicted to Sugar

In This Chapter

▶ Understanding why sugar is so addictive

▶ Investigating different kinds of addicts

*I*n addition to being the driving force behind a multitude of health problems, sugar is a powerful, mood-altering substance that's as addictive as cocaine (more on that later in this chapter). No other food component affects your brain as strongly as sugar, and many people literally become addicted to the effects it has on their brain chemistry.

Humans are prone to sugar addiction for many reasons. Everyone has a genetic predisposition to seek out the sweet stuff, and sugar (especially the processed kind) exerts strong effects on the brain and body chemistry that keep people hooked. Many people learn unhealthy eating cues and habits from their parents, and modern society makes sugar plentiful, cheap, and enticing. My goal for this book is to help you gain control over your eating, your health, and your life!

In this chapter, I explore why sugar is so addictive and give you a glimpse into the behavior and psychology of four typical types of sugar addicts. You can take a quiz for each type of sugar addict to see how closely you resemble the common profile and then follow the advice I give for each kind.

Getting to the Root of Why Sugar Is So Darned Addictive

Sugar addiction is prevalent in modern society because sugar is legal, cheap, pervasive, and socially acceptable. You can't say that about the other substances people get addicted to. Combine all that with a stressful job, a harried family life, and an impossible schedule, and is it any wonder that people stuff themselves with sugar-packed convenience foods?

But sugar's addictiveness isn't just a matter of social acceptance and availability. Sugar is physically addictive, affecting both the body and the brain. In this section, I cover some of the physical, emotional, and social reasons why sugar is so addictive.

Brain chemistry

Sugar (along with its addiction-prone cousins, starch, salt, and fat) is one of the stimulating foodstuffs termed *hyperpalatables* — foods that stimulate the pleasure centers in the brain. Central to the brain's sensation of enjoyment is a chemical called *dopamine,* a neurotransmitter that controls the brain's reward and pleasure centers. When you eat sugar, it stimulates a dopamine release, and you experience a pleasurable sensation. It's easy for humans to get hooked on dopamine and consequently become addicted to the things that produce it — sugar, alcohol, cocaine, sex, methamphetamines, and so on.

Science shows that sugar acts on your brain's reward system just like cocaine. That's right, to your brain, the mountain of frosting on that cupcake is just like crack. As with any dopamine-producing substance, your brain gets desensitized to it with chronic overconsumption, and you develop a tolerance. That means that to create the pleasurable feeling, you have to use more and more. This launches a vicious cycle of increased consumption leading to further desensitization, and you end up with an insatiable appetite for sugar (or whatever other substance you're abusing).

Making matters more difficult, science has shown that as dopamine receptors decrease, there's a marked decrease in the activity of the *prefrontal cortex* — the part of your brain responsible for "executive" functions like planning, organizing, and making rational decisions. This is a double-whammy for the sugar addict — not only do you have to eat more sugar to experience the normal reward and pleasure, but your addiction also makes it more difficult for your brain to plan ahead and make sensible food decisions!

Genetic programming

Humans are programmed to crave high-energy foods. Back in the cave man days, high-calorie foods meant a high chance of survival, so you're genetically programmed to prefer high-calorie foods (fat and sugar) over all others.

Dopamine desires: Losing a sense of reason

Dopamine does more than just kick out pleasure signals. This neurotransmitter affects brain processes that control voluntary movement, emotional responses, motivation, and the ability to anticipate rewards. Dopamine deficiency results in Parkinson's disease and has also been implicated in schizophrenia, ADHD, and restless leg syndrome. Studies show that people with low dopamine activity appear to be more prone to addiction, and the presence of a certain kind of dopamine receptor is associated with sensation-seeking (addict) or thrill-seeking (adrenaline junkie) behavior.

The feelings of satisfaction that dopamine exerts are so strong that, to obtain that satisfaction, an addict often loses the ability to reason. Because the brain develops neural circuits that unconsciously assess reward, addicts will do what they think is in their best interest, when in fact the only interest such behavior satisfies is the release of dopamine. The unconscious need for the release of dopamine becomes all-important to the junkie, and consequences and reason fly out the window.

Exercise not only improves the functioning of the prefrontal cortex but also directly regenerates dopamine receptors, helping to both rebuild the damage of past addiction and prevent it in the future! See Chapter 12 for exercise tips.

Over the last few years, some fascinating research has come to light in the field of *epigenetics* — the study of the body's chemistry that switches genes off and on. Not surprisingly, your diet and your environment change your body chemistry, and scientists are learning how this affects the switching on and off of certain genes that affect how your body processes food.

Here's a great example of a lifestyle that changes your gene expression to your detriment: You wake up already tired, hit the snooze button a few times, skip breakfast, and fly out the door after yelling at your kids and feeling awful about how fat you look in your outfit. Then you spend most of your day sitting glued to a computer screen in a stressed-out, fight-or-flight overdrive, trying to meet some deadline given to you by someone who doesn't understand you and who doesn't care that you're surrounded by people who are just making your job harder. To anesthetize the pain of this stressed-out existence and to quiet the part of your brain that's screaming for fuel, you grab whatever junk food is easily obtained nearby. This constant dependence on the quick sugar fix not only thickens your waistline but also changes your gene expression to one that supports fat storage and addiction. As Aristotle said, "We are what we repeatedly do."

Your DNA is not your destiny! You can't alter the genes you were born with, but you *can* change which of those genes express themselves by modifying how you eat and how you live. As you start to eat better and lead a healthier lifestyle, your gene expression will change to reflect the improvements in your body chemistry.

Feeding yeast infections

A yeast infection is an overgrowth of one or more of the naturally occurring fungi (typically the *Candida albicans* yeast) that inhabit dark, moist parts of your body. Your immune system usually keeps *Candida* from growing out of control, but if the immune system is compromised, an overgrowth can occur.

A high-sugar diet lowers your immune system's power (see Chapter 4 for more on the immune system) and reduces the amount of beneficial bacteria in your intestines (which further weakens the immune system). Yeast feeds on sugar, and yeast grows best in an acidic environment. Eating lots of sugar gives the yeast both of those conditions.

Because yeast feeds on sugar, it typically triggers very strong cravings for sugar (and sometimes alcohol). This starts a vicious cycle; the more sugar you eat, the more yeast grows, and the stronger the cravings become.

Antibiotic use kills off the beneficial bacteria in your intestines (the *intestinal flora*), giving yeast and other opportunistic microorganisms a big "Vacancy" sign. After a course of antibiotics, it's important to replace the beneficial bacteria with a good probiotic supplement (see Chapter 5 for the scoop on probiotics).

Frequent or persistent yeast infections that go untreated can damage the intestines, overtax the immune system, cause systemic inflammation, and spread to other organs and tissues. If you're prone to yeast infections, you need to change to a low-sugar diet immediately and begin an aggressive course of probiotic therapy. Consult a knowledgeable healthcare practitioner for guidance, and if he gives you an antibiotic or antifungal medication and sends you on your way without any discussion of diet and probiotics, seek out a better practitioner (see Chapter 7 for some healthcare practitioner advice).

Hunger and cravings

Leptin is a hormone that signals to your brain that you've had enough to eat, producing a sensation of fullness (satiety). Leptin is produced in the fat cells, so the more fat you have, the more leptin you produce. This is nature's way of keeping your weight under control. If you eat a normal, healthy diet, this system works fine, but an unhealthy lifestyle can easily screw up the natural leptin-signaling system.

Nature's "full" signal can get disrupted by many things, such as carrying too much body fat, maintaining chronically high insulin levels, ingesting too many artificial sweeteners, consuming excess sugar (especially fructose), or having elevated triglycerides. When your leptin signals fail (a condition called *leptin resistance*), your hunger hormones run rampant and unopposed. This is why a consistent sugar overload, even though it fills you with calories and raises your blood sugar levels, stimulates hunger and cravings.

To reverse the hunger-hormone tailspin that a high-sugar diet creates, you need to eat foods that promote satiety (protein, fibrous vegetables, nuts, and seeds) and avoid foods that raise insulin (sugar, fructose, sweetened drinks, and processed grain). Both exercise and weight loss boost the effectiveness and sensitivity of insulin and leptin.

Learned behavior

Humans are creatures of habit. Food preferences start early in life, and after children develop the habit of eating sugar, fat, and salt, they get locked into a self-perpetuating cycle of preferring these foods into adulthood (scientists call this *pervasive palate preference*). Your love affair with sugar probably started at an early age. As a child, your parents or grandparents may have given you sweets as a reward or as a distraction to calm you down. As an adult, this naturally becomes an emotional crutch if you still equate sugar with being good or being calm.

Associating certain events with sugar is another thing that most people learn over their lifetimes. Cake is typically a centerpiece of birthdays, weddings, retirement parties, and the like. Holiday celebrations such as Easter, Rosh Hashanah, Halloween, Thanksgiving, and Christmas often revolve around sweets. See Chapter 10 for tips on surviving holidays and special occasions.

Many addicts learn to reach for sugar as an attempt to avoid negative feelings like stress, loneliness, or low self-esteem. These habits quickly become destructive, addictive behaviors as you learn to use a sugar coma to squelch genuine emotions that desperately need your attention.

Polite conventions in society tend to perpetuate sugar abuse. If you have people over to your house for dinner, you naturally assume you have to serve them dessert too, right? And as the guest, you feel obligated to eat it even if you don't want it because you don't want to appear rude. Offering a heroin needle to your guests would be bizarre, but offering (and accepting) sugar appears to be obligatory.

By using the techniques in this book to change how you view sugar and how you plan your food, you can unlearn the unhealthy programming, remain aware of your triggers, and stay in control of your own behavior.

What Kind of Sweet Freak Are You?

The following sections outline the four main types of sugar addicts and explain some general behavior and psychology traits common to each one. If you understand what kind of sugar addict you are and you learn to recognize some behaviors and thought patterns common to each addict type, you may start to understand how you've become addicted to sugar. Even more important, you'll discover what you need to do to overcome your addiction and regain control of your life.

Answer the questions for each quiz using the following scoring system:

0 points for "Never"

2 points for "Sometimes, but rarely"

5 points for "Half the time"

10 points for "Most of the time" or "Always"

If you'd like more information to help you evaluate whether you're addicted to sugar, turn to Chapter 1.

The Exhausted Addict

To determine how closely you resemble the classic Exhausted Addict, take the following quiz using the scoring system at the beginning of this section.

_____ Do you need caffeine to get started in the morning or to make it through the day?

_____ Do you have trouble going to sleep, or do you wake up in the middle of the night without being able to go back to sleep?

_____ Do you crave sweets when you get tired?

_____ Do you experience indigestion or acid reflux?

_____ Do you feel like you're always running — that there are never enough hours in the day?

_____ Do you have chronic aches, pains, and tight muscles?

_____ Do you get headaches?

_____ Do you put others' needs above your own?

_____ Do you think that if you don't do it, it won't get done?

_____ Do you eat sugar or fast food because you don't have time for something healthy?

Now add up your score:

0–30 points: You don't show strong signs of being an Exhausted Addict.

31–50 points: You exhibit some of the Exhausted Addict symptoms. Chances are you'll score similarly for at least one other type of addict.

51–100 points: You fit the mold of the classic Exhausted Addict. Read on and see whether the following description of the typical Exhausted Addict's personality sounds like you.

Understanding the Exhausted Addict

If you're an Exhausted Addict, you're the epitome of someone who runs herself too hard. You don't know the meaning of the word *downtime,* and fatigue is almost constant. There never seem to be enough hours in the day to get everything done, and you pressure yourself to try to be the one who does everything for everyone except yourself.

Exhausted Addicts are generally perfectionists who can't accept anything except the best from themselves. They see themselves as the go-to person when a crisis arises, and they create an unhealthy sense of pride by ignoring their own self-care and putting everyone else's needs before theirs.

Exhausted Addicts regularly have sore muscles, trigger points, and areas that stay tight and painful. Stress and poor breathing habits keep muscles tight and turned on when they shouldn't be. Painful knots and trigger points develop, and with an overactive nervous system, this can progress to a chronic pain condition known as *fibromyalgia* (see Chapter 4).

Due to stresses (both external and self-created), marginal diet, and lack of sleep, the Exhausted Addict's adrenal function becomes impaired (see Chapter 4). This is referred to as *adrenal fatigue,* and it results in chronic fatigue, low thyroid function, and low blood sugar that triggers sugar cravings.

Exhausted Addicts tend to eat poorly because they think planning their eating requires too much time and attention. Instead of sitting down for a healthy meal, these types of addicts grab whatever's handy, often turning to sugar or other junk food to give them the energy boost they desperately need.

The stress from the Exhausted Addict's punishing schedule causes insomnia and restless sleep. Lack of sleep disrupts the normal production of appetite-suppressing hormones, so the Exhausted Addict is prone to hunger and cravings. If you reach for the sugar when this happens, you'll find that, like most other addicts of this type, you can no longer fit in your skinny jeans.

Advice for the Exhausted Addict

In addition to weaning yourself off sugar with the techniques in Part III, you can benefit from learning to *plan* instead of *react.* Because your life feels so out of control and pressured, any amount of preplanned control helps reduce your stress levels and improve your eating. See Chapter 8 for tips on planning and eating mindfully instead of reactively.

The Sad Eater

To determine how closely you resemble the classic Sad Eater, take the following quiz using the scoring system at the beginning of this section.

_____ Are you lonely?

_____ Do you find yourself wishing your life were drastically different?

_____ Do you have a decreased sex drive?

_____ Do you tend to do the same things week in and week out?

_____ Do you have strong PMS symptoms?

_____ Do you turn to sugar or other comfort foods when you feel sad or lonely?

_____ Do you wake up tired no matter how long you've slept?

_____ Do you gossip or talk about others behind their back? Be honest!

_____ Do you feel depressed or hopeless?

_____ Do you eat sugar late at night, regardless of whether you're hungry or not?

Now tally up your score:

> 0–25 points: You don't show strong signs of being a Sad Eater.
>
> 26–50 points: You exhibit some of the Sad Eater symptoms. Chances are you'll score similarly for at least one other type of addict.
>
> 51–100 points: You fit the mold of the classic Sad Eater. Read on and see whether the following description of the typical Sad Eater's personality sounds like you.

Understanding the Sad Eater

As the name implies, Sad Eaters spend a lot of time feeling sad and depressed. They use sugar as an artificial mood elevator, and their behaviors with food embody the very definition of the term _emotional eater._ Out of all the addict types, the Sad Eater has the unhealthiest relationship with food. It's common for Sad Eaters to turn to sugar for comfort and companionship; often Sad Eaters feel like food is their only friend, even if they're surrounded by family or co-workers.

Sad Eaters often have a strong _inner critic_ (see Chapter 9), with self-esteem problems stemming from childhood. Many Sad Eaters find themselves in a difficult Catch-22 with food — they feel fat and unlovable, so they eat sugar for comfort, telling themselves they "just don't care." A high-sugar diet, of course, leads to more body fat and a worse self-image, feeding both the fat cells and the pity party.

Sad eaters often act angry, crabby, and/or judgmental toward others. If you find yourself regularly getting irritated with co-workers or angry with family members because they don't act according to your expectations, you may be exhibiting Sad Eater behavior.

Sad Eaters are commonly perimenopausal or are particularly sensitive to PMS and monthly hormone fluctuations. Hormone deficiencies and imbalances can wreak havoc with their emotional state. If you have a deficiency of estrogen, progesterone, and/or testosterone, you can become sad or even clinically depressed. When this happens, you start to crave sugar in an attempt to raise your serotonin levels (see Chapter 4 for more on serotonin).

Advice for the Sad Eater

If you're a Sad Eater, you can more easily stay away from sugar if you develop a better sense of emotional awareness. Do some self-inquiry to uncover more details about the negative emotions that you're experiencing — the more specific the better. For example, if you're feeling stressed at work, try to find some more accurate and specific words to describe what you're feeling. Instead of just stressed, do you feel overwhelmed? Unappreciated? Afraid? Trapped? Inadequate? When you start to understand a more detailed picture of your reactions and emotions, you're able to more accurately assess the situation and deal with the truth instead of just reacting negatively and reaching for the sugar.

Some professional therapy may help steer you toward greater emotional awareness. See Chapter 11 for tips on seeking out support groups and professional help.

In addition to weaning yourself off sugar with the tools in Part III, you need to put extra effort and attention on the substitute behaviors covered in Chapter 9. The best things to boost your mood are to do something outside the normal routine and to do something good for someone else.

The Undereater

To determine how closely you resemble the classic Undereater, take the following quiz using the scoring system at the beginning of this section.

_____ Are you tired most of the day?

_____ When something stressful happens to you, does your energy nose-dive?

_____ Do you skip breakfast?

_____ Do you eat a low-protein diet (only one or two protein servings per day)? See Chapter 5 if you're not sure what constitutes a serving of protein.

_____ Do you have cravings at night?

_____ Do you drink less than eight glasses of water per day?

_____ Do you eat a most of your food for the day after 5 p.m.?

_____ Do you need caffeine to stay alert in the middle of the day?

_____ Do you have trouble concentrating?

_____ Do you get irritable with people?

Now tally up your score:

0–25 points: You don't show signs of being a classic Undereater.

26–45 points: You exhibit some signs of being an Undereater. Chances are you'll score similarly for at least one other type of addict.

46–100 points: You definitely fit the mold of the classic Undereater. Read on and see whether the following description of the typical Undereater's personality sounds like yours.

Understanding the Undereater

Classic Undereaters are often low-energy people. They love to sleep, and they generally find it very difficult to muster the energy to do anything above and beyond what is absolutely necessary — even things they enjoy. In that respect, Undereaters are similar to Exhausted Addicts (discussed earlier in this section), but while Exhausted Addicts continue to unhealthily push themselves through their stress and exhaustion, Undereaters crash and shut down instead.

If you're an Undereater, you probably have a history of spinning your wheels and feeling stuck or trapped in your job, your family issues, and your body size. You may often feel out of touch with others and regularly ignore your own emotional problems, admitting that "I just can't deal with that right now."

You seldom eat breakfast, and when you do, it's usually an all-carb affair. In fact, most of your food is carbohydrate. You tell yourself that you eat enough protein "on most days," but if you journal your food for a few days, you'll see that you barely eat one or two servings of protein a day — not even enough to meet the recommended daily intake, let alone enough to be healthy and energetic. Eating like this keeps your metabolism low, so you probably find yourself gaining weight even though you don't eat much.

Like many sugar addicts, you probably feel overwhelmed with making food choices. You've tried dozens of frustrating diets and special detoxes over the years, none of which has yielded any long-term success. Eating healthy takes too much thinking and planning, so like the Exhausted Addict, you turn to sugar because it's easy.

Advice for the Undereater

By beginning to wean yourself off sugar, you'll start to feel more energetic and feel like you have more control over your food choices. In addition to following the how-to advice in Part III of this book, the best advice I have for Undereaters is as follows:

- ✔ Make sure you eat protein at every meal.
- ✔ When you have a sugar craving, get up and *do* something! Your body and your brain are craving activity and stimulation, so take a walk, write in your journal, or do some sit-ups instead of continuing to drug yourself with sugar!

The Sugar Stalker

To determine how closely you resemble the classic Sugar Stalker, take the following quiz using the scoring system at the beginning of this section.

_____ Do you keep a stash of sweets at work or in the pantry at home?

_____ Do you drink sweetened drinks?

_____ Do you get headaches or become irritable if you skip your sugar fix?

_____ Do you eat sweet things like pastries or donuts first thing in the day?

_____ When you start eating sugar, do you have trouble stopping?

_____ Do you have a craving for something sweet after every meal?

_____ Do you become stressed when you think about changing your eating habits?

_____ Are you a chocoholic?

_____ Do you hide sweets or are you embarrassed to eat them in front of others?

_____ Do you order dessert at a restaurant even if you're full?

Now add up your score:

0–30 points: You don't show strong signs of being a Sugar Stalker.

31–50 points: You exhibit some of the Sugar Stalker symptoms. Chances are you'll score similarly for at least one other type of addict.

51–100 points: You behave like the classic Sugar Stalker. Read on and see whether the following description of the typical Sugar Stalker sounds like you.

Understanding the Sugar Stalker

Out of all the addicts, the Sugar Stalker is most physically addicted to sugar — meaning true chemical/physiological addiction. The Sugar Stalker's taste buds have been overstimulated and desensitized to the point of finding nothing but the most over-sugared, sickly sweet treats to be even remotely satisfying.

If you're a Sugar Stalker, your life revolves around sugar to the point where your eyes light up and your mouth starts to water at the very mention of something sweet. Sugar Stalkers eat a stream of sugar throughout the day, starting with a high-sugar breakfast of sweetened coffee, pastries, or fruit juice. Sweet snacks like candies and cookies are the norm, and the thought of drinking something that isn't sweetened — even water — turns their stomach.

Sugar Stalkers, like many people addicted to a given substance, act impulsively when presented with their object of addiction. They can't say no when offered something sweet and have a hard time knowing when to say when.

Interestingly, Sugar Stalkers are very often shy, introverted people despite the outward appearance of being very social and having many friends. Many suffer from self-esteem problems even though they display a bubbly personality on the outside.

Advice for the Sugar Stalker

If you're a Sugar Stalker, you need to quit sweetened drinks cold turkey. Your taste buds and the dopamine reward center in your brain need to be re-sensitized to what normal food tastes like, and sweet drinks — even diet sodas with no actual sugar — make that impossible. See Chapter 9 for ideas for substitute beverages and for a step-by-step flowchart of what to do when a sugar craving strikes.

In addition to becoming a disciple of Chapter 9, you need to redefine dessert. To gradually disengage from the habit of having to have something sweet after every meal, start substituting sweet things that are healthier — a few berries or grapes instead of cake, for example. My personal favorite is a few bites of sharp cheddar or havarti cheese and a strawberry.

Portion control is another thing that helps you get off sugar (see Chapter 5 for more on portion control). If you're a Sugar Stalker, it's important for you to apportion your healthier sweets so you're not tempted to keep eating. Never eat from a package; put your allowance on a plate instead, and that's all you get. Two bites are all that most people need to be satisfied — any more just adds extra calories without extra satisfaction. Try one piece (and only one!) of dark chocolate or maltitol-sweetened, sugar-free chocolate, and let it melt in your mouth for a long time.

Chapter 3

The 4-1-1 on Sugar and Carbs

Your body doesn't deal with all carbohydrates in the same fashion. Different types of carbs have different effects on your body chemistry. Overcoming your sugar addiction requires the ability to evaluate carbohydrates and an understanding of how the choices you make affect your body.

Information about sugar and low-carb eating can be confusing, so this chapter delivers the lowdown on carbohydrates and sugars, how your body processes them, and how you can distinguish good carbs from bad carbs.

To make a responsible nutrition plan, recognizing where your sugar intake comes from is important. This chapter discusses some common sources of dietary sugar, including many hidden sources of which you may not be aware.

One of the common techniques for attempting to reduce carbohydrate intake is to eliminate gluten from the diet. Though gluten doesn't have anything to do with sugar addiction, some people have an easier time cutting back on their total carb intake if they stop eating wheat. So I dedicate a section of this chapter to guiding you through the basic principles of going gluten-free.

Finally, I include important information here for you and your loved ones — the shocking truth about the dangers of artificial sweeteners.

Sugar: The New Poison

The epidemic of obesity and diabetes in the Western world has three main causes: the sugar content in food, inactivity, and increased overall calorie consumption. Combining all three, as has happened over the years, creates the perfect storm for a health and wellness catastrophe.

Sugar abuse can lead to a myriad of health problems, including weight gain, diabetes, depressed immunity, elevated cholesterol and triglycerides, cancer, tooth decay, yeast infections, liver disease, depression, chronic fatigue, increased appetite, and metabolic syndrome. If a pharmaceutical company put a pill on the drugstore shelves that could cause all those side effects, an outcry would ensue, followed by quick action to get the pill removed from the public's reach!

But sugar is a food product, even though it has drug-like effects. It's cheap, it's abundant, and people *love it.* Sugar is pervasive in our society, and therein lies the problem.

As of this writing, sugar consumption in the United States has risen to approximately 130 pounds per person every year. That's almost 650 calories of added sugar every day! The average American drinks a staggering *53 gallons* of soft drinks per year. Americans consume ten times more sugar than any other food additive.

The biggest culprits in the Western food supply are sweetened beverages, candy, and baked goods. Those account for approximately three-fourths of the total sugar that people consume. So by cutting out junk food like that, you can easily reduce your sugar consumption by 75 percent!

The Science of Carbohydrates

Carbohydrates — you hear and read the word all the time. Good carbs, bad carbs, low-carb, high-carb, sugary carbs — what does it all mean?

In a nutshell, a *carbohydrate* is any one of a group of compounds that includes sugars, starches, and cellulose (fiber). Your body digests the carbohydrates that you eat and breaks them down into a sugar called *glucose,* which is the preferred form of carbohydrate that the body uses for fuel.

Identifying sources of carbohydrates

Many folks mistakenly think of carbohydrates as only starches (pasta, bread, potatoes, and so on) and sweets. But you find carbs in a variety of other foods. Here's a quick list of dietary sources of carbohydrates:

- ✔ Fruits
- ✔ Grain products like breads, cereals, and pastas
- ✔ Sugars like candy, honey, sweetened beverages, syrups, and table sugar
- ✔ Vegetables

A good rule of thumb is that if it grows in the ground, it contains carbohydrates. A few exceptions exist — like peanuts, which are higher in fat and protein than they are in carbohydrates — but for the most part, if it's a plant or if it's made from a plant, it's mostly carbohydrate.

Seeing why sugar is so bad for you

Carbohydrates are very important to living beings. You need carbohydrates in your diet to provide energy to each cell, to supply your brain with glucose, and to furnish fuel for your muscles and organs. All your DNA and RNA molecules have a sugar molecule (ribose) in them. In fact, if you don't eat enough carbohydrates, your body breaks down muscle tissue to make some!

So if carbohydrates are so important, why is sugar so bad for you? What's with all the low-carb buzz?

The physiological response you get from eating any carbohydrate depends on the *type* of carb and the *amount* that you eat. Do it right and you have a normal, healthy response. Do it wrong and the chemistry created in your body makes you fat, sick, and addicted.

Here are the basic steps of what happens to the carbohydrates that you eat:

1. **Your digestive system breaks down carbohydrates (first in your mouth with saliva and chewing, and then from digestive enzymes in your small intestine) into smaller bits of carbohydrate known as *monosaccharides*.**

2. **Your liver absorbs the monosaccharides and, like a dispatcher, sends them out to do various important jobs — feed the brain, make cells to do their thing, and fill up your muscles and organs with fuel.**

3. **After these jobs are finished, your body promptly packages up and stores any leftover carbs as body fat.**

Note: Hereafter I use the word *sugar* to mean a food that is a low-nutrient, fiber-free carbohydrate like candy, high-fructose corn syrup, sugared soda, and table sugar, even though other types of carbohydrates are technically broken down into sugars too.

The problem with sugar is that it's not only high in calories but also virtually nutrient- and fiber-free. When you eat a lot of sugar (especially without fiber, protein, or fat), far too much sugar enters the bloodstream at one time. This creates a chemical emergency in your body, which responds to the assault by prompting the pancreas to release a large dose of insulin to attempt to control the sugar levels.

Connecting carbs and sugar to insulin

Diabetes is one of the biggest threats to modern human health. With high sugar intake, low amounts of exercise, and too many calories overall (which unfortunately describes most of America these days), the body is forced to produce more and more *insulin,* a hormone that's essential for preventing a dangerous buildup of sugar in your bloodstream but that, at high levels, can cause problems.

High insulin levels cause you to store fat and crave more food. This cycle continues over the years, and as you gain weight, your body becomes less and less sensitive to insulin, and it craves more and more sugar. The end result is obesity and insulin resistance, which lead to diabetes. (Chapter 4 tells you more about diabetes and other health problems linked to sugar.)

The most important source of fuel for your body is glucose, which enters the bloodstream after you eat. Glucose then travels throughout your bloodstream and is used by every cell in your body for energy.

The pancreas, an organ located behind your stomach, is in charge of releasing hormones that make your body either store or release calories. One of those hormones is insulin.

Insulin "unlocks" your cells to allow the sugar circulating in the blood to enter the cells, where it can be turned into energy. After you eat a meal, your pancreas senses a rise in your blood sugar level and releases the insulin needed to move sugar from your blood into your cells. When you eat too many carbohydrates (especially sugars and low-fiber carbs), your pancreas is forced to secrete a lot of insulin to manage all that sugar.

Insulin generally does an adequate job of shuttling all that sugar to the right places (including turning all the extra sugar into fat), but regularly having high insulin levels causes several serious problems:

✔ High insulin levels decrease your ability to burn body fat for fuel.

✔ Over time your body becomes less sensitive to all the extra insulin, and it requires more and more of it to control blood sugar levels. This is called *insulin resistance,* and it inevitably leads to type 2 diabetes.

✔ High insulin levels lower blood sugar levels — that's insulin's job, after all. Too much insulin lowers blood sugar levels too far. Sugar crash! This causes more cravings.

✔ High insulin levels make you sleepy and sluggish.

Selecting Desirable Carbs versus Undesirable Carbs

Not all carbohydrates are the same, and despite what some mainstream diets pronounce, not every carbohydrate is your enemy. Now that you understand how insulin works (see the preceding section), it's time to discover how to select carbohydrates that give you a slow release of glucose into the body.

Separating complex carbs from simple carbs

As a general rule, the more stuff the digestive system has to break down, the more gradual the sugar release into the bloodstream is. Slower is better because a slower sugar release means you produce less insulin. For healthy insulin response, you should choose carbohydrates that are *complex* — carbs that are made up of long chains of sugar molecules and therefore take longer to break down. Examples of complex carbohydrates are fibrous vegetables like greens and beans and whole-grain starches like brown rice, quinoa, and whole wheat.

To further slow down sugar release, try to eat protein and fat with those complex carbohydrates!

Simple carbohydrates consist of only one or two molecules and thus break down and enter the bloodstream very quickly. This makes the pancreas release a lot of insulin to control the rapid rise in sugar levels. High insulin levels cause a lot of problems, so try to stay away from simple carbs. Simple carbohydrates are sugars and sweet stuff like candy, corn syrup, fruit juice, powdered sugar, sweetened beverages, and table sugar.

A more accurate representation of the speed of a carbohydrate's entry into the bloodstream is the *glycemic load,* which I discuss in Chapter 5.

Getting more fiber and nutrition per calorie

The best kind of carbohydrates are the ones that contain lots of fiber, are relatively low in calories, and have high nutrient content per calorie. So generally, fibrous vegetables fit the bill nicely.

A good rule of thumb is that the darker a vegetable or grain is, the more nutrients it contains. Dark, leafy greens are more nutritious than white iceberg lettuce. Quinoa, brown rice, and wild rice have more nutrients than white rice.

Most of your carbohydrates should come from vegetables because they're high in nutrients and low in calories. Their glycemic load (see Chapter 5 for the scoop on glycemic load) is low, so you can eat a large volume of vegetables without consuming too many total carbohydrates.

To make a global statement, you can pretty much eat all the vegetables you want without getting into too much trouble.

If you have gastrointestinal issues like Crohn's disease or irritable bowel syndrome (IBS), you may need to temper the amount of fiber you consume. Readers with these medical conditions should consult a qualified professional for personalized advice.

Fruits are high in nutrition, but they're also higher in calories and sugar (fructose) than vegetables, so be judicious in your consumption. Avoid drinking fruit juice because it's basically fiber-free and very high in calories and sugar.

Addressing problems with fructose

As I mention earlier in the chapter, not all carbohydrates are the same. A particular kind of sugar called *fructose* is particularly troublesome in the Western diet.

Fructose occurs naturally in fruit. From that source it generally isn't a problem because, in natural foods, fructose is bound to glucose, so you don't eat that much of it (and that's as complicated as I need to get for the purposes of this lesson).

However, fructose is also prevalent as a sweetener (agave nectar, crystalline fructose, high-fructose corn syrup, honey, and so on), and that becomes a biological problem. Humans can digest only a small amount of fructose. Eating too much fructose can cause bloating, flatulence, and loose stools.

What about alcohol?

Alcoholic drinks generally contain only small amounts of sugar (assuming that you don't add lots of sugary mixer). Even a glass of sweet white wine usually contains only about 8 grams of sugar. But be careful — this doesn't mean that the wine is low in total carbohydrates or calories! Most alcoholic beverages consist of mostly high-glycemic carbohydrates.

Despite its relatively low sugar content, alcohol can have a drastic effect on your blood sugar levels. Although alcohol may cause a slight rise in blood sugar levels when you initially ingest it, the overall effect of alcohol is to cause a drop in blood sugar. The more you drink, the more your blood sugar drops. Drinking as little as 2 ounces of alcohol on an empty stomach can lead to a very low blood sugar level, which can be a big problem for anyone with diabetes. It also increases your appetite, as anyone who has had too much to drink can attest to.

Over time, excessive alcohol consumption can decrease insulin's effectiveness, resulting in high blood sugar levels and insulin resistance. One study showed that 70 percent of people with alcoholic liver disease had either glucose intolerance or diabetes.

Food manufacturers have recently begun using sugar alcohols as sweeteners. *Sugar alcohols* are technically neither sugars nor alcohols; they're carbohydrates with a chemical structure that partially resembles sugar and partially resembles alcohol (but they don't contain ethanol, like alcoholic beverages do). *Polyols,* as sugar alcohols are also known, aren't completely absorbed and metabolized by the body and consequently contribute about 25 percent fewer calories than most sugars — but you should still consider them sugar. Many sugar alcohols have unpleasant side effects, including bloating, stomach cramps, and diarrhea. Commonly used sugar alcohols include erythritol, isomalt, lactitol, maltitol, maltitol syrup, mannitol, sorbitol, and xylitol.

Overconsumption of fructose is also a major factor in weight gain. The process of digestion breaks down most carbohydrates into glucose, which is the most basic fuel on the planet. All your cells use it, so your body processes it efficiently because it goes literally everywhere in the body. Fructose, however, is a very different simple sugar that isn't used in cells. All fructose goes to the liver, where most of it is immediately converted into triglycerides (fat). When you consistently eat a lot of fructose, you not only overload your liver (causing fatty liver disease) but also basically create body fat on the spot.

Here are some more problems with consuming large amounts of fructose:

- ✔ **Cardiovascular problems:** Excess fructose in the diet causes elevated cholesterol, homocysteine, and triglyceride levels.

- ✔ **Leptin insensitivity:** Fructose doesn't stimulate the production of *leptin,* an appetite-suppressing hormone, like other carbohydrates do. The brain, unable to recognize that leptin is present, responds as if the body is starving. It then signals the body to lower the rate of metabolism and to store any fat that happens to be in the food. Hence, a high-fructose diet leads to extra storage of dietary fat and increased appetite.

✔ **Toxic byproducts:** The liver's metabolism of fructose creates a long list of waste products and toxins, including a large amount of uric acid, which increases blood pressure and can cause gout.

According to the *American Journal of Clinical Nutrition,* corn syrup sweeteners now represent more than 20 percent of total daily carbohydrate intake for the average American. Don't be average!

Current research shows that approximately half of the population is unable to digest 25 grams of fructose by itself. Naturally occurring fructose (found in fruits) is bound with glucose, making absorption a non-issue in reasonable amounts. Processed fructose (like high-fructose corn syrup and crystalline fructose) is a different story. This type of sugar can easily overload the liver. You should limit your consumption of fructose (especially the artificial kind!), and if you have to eat it, don't exceed 25 grams.

Making substitutions for better carbs and less sugar

One of the easiest things you can do to reduce your sugar intake and keep your insulin levels under control is to substitute healthier carbohydrates for the ones containing more sugar and less fiber.

Table 3-1 can help you make some smart substitutions in your day-to-day food decisions.

Table 3-1   Substituting Smarter Carbs for Sugary Carbs

Instead of This	Eat This
White pasta	Brown rice pasta
	Whole-wheat pasta
Fruit juice	Green tea
Coffee with sugar	Coffee with stevia
Jelly	Strawberry slices
	Blueberries
Corn flakes	Slow-cooked oatmeal

Instead of This	Eat This
Soda	Mineral water with citrus slices
Candy	Dark chocolate (minimum 70% cacao)
After-dinner sweet	Chewing gum or breath mint
White bread	Whole-grain bread (and half the amount!)
White rice	Quinoa
	Brown rice
Midafternoon junk food	Crunchy raw vegetables
Breakfast sweet roll or muffin	One slice of whole-grain toast topped with scrambled egg
Commercial trail mix	Handful of almonds
Pie	Apple slices with cheese
Pudding	Cottage cheese
Cake	One slice of whole-grain cinnamon-raisin or cranberry toast with butter or low-fat cream cheese
Ice cream	Non-GMO popcorn (popped yourself, not commercial microwave "popcorn" in a bag)

It's important to read the labels on prepared or packaged foods because what may seem like a healthy choice may be the opposite. For example, many commercial trail mixes are loaded with sugar and chemicals, and bread with "whole wheat" on the package may not truly be whole wheat. Flip to Chapter 6 for more info about reading labels.

Understanding Where Your Sugar Intake Comes From

Knowing the facts about carbohydrates and insulin response gives you a good idea of which carbs to eat and which to stay away from. This section goes into more detail about the sugar content of common foods and ways you can identify hidden sources of sugar from food labels (more on successfully deciphering food labels in Chapter 6).

A good rule of thumb is to stay away from any prepared food that has more than 10 grams of sugar per serving. That's a decent benchmark for evaluating the overall sugariness of a food.

When you start paying attention to the nutrition facts of some common foods, you may very well be surprised that foods generally considered to be healthy — such as dried fruit, vitamin water, and 100-percent fruit juice — often have far more sugar than things you consider dessert!

Picking out obvious sources of sugar

When considering foods to stay away from, the obvious sugary treats are the easiest to identify:

- ✔ Candy (yes, that means milk chocolate)
- ✔ Cookies, donuts, and other sugary baked goods
- ✔ Sugared beverages like soda and sweet tea
- ✔ Sweetened breakfast cereals

When you investigate the labels of the foods in your pantry and refrigerator, some of the common sources of sugar will be obvious — anything that says *sugar* or *syrup* is a dead giveaway. And that means give it away!

You can read all about cleaning out and restocking your kitchen in Chapter 6.

Uncovering hidden sources of sugar

Many foods that are generally considered healthy are actually quite high in sugar content. That doesn't mean that they don't have nutritional value, but it does mean that you have to be aware of how much sugar they contain. Orange juice isn't bad for you, for example, but it does have a lot of sugar and a lot of calories in one small glass. So drink it sparingly.

Here are some common foods, drinks, and condiments whose sugar content may surprise you:

- ✔ **Bottled teas:** Tea is good for you, right? Yes, but unless you make it yourself, it may be packed with sugar and other unhealthy ingredients. A 20-ounce bottle of SoBe Green Tea has . . . wait for it . . . 51 grams of sugar!

- ✔ **Children's drinks:** One Hi-C Flashin' Fruit Punch juice box contains only 10 percent real juice, with 30 grams of sugar and lots of chemicals.

- ✔ **Coffee drinks:** A Starbucks grande Caffè Vanilla Frappuccino (16 ounces) weighs in at a whopping 58 grams of sugar!

- ✔ **Dried fruit:** A small handful (⅓ cup) of dried cranberries has 26 grams of sugar. Seven pieces of Wild Garden dried apricots contain 21 grams of sugar.

- ✔ **Energy bars and snack bars:** Several of the best-selling energy bars are nothing more than glorified candy bars. Just because it has a picture of granola or an athlete on the wrapper doesn't mean it's a high-quality snack.

- **Energy drinks:** Most energy drinks consist of caffeine, sugar, and a high dose of B vitamins to give you a buzz for an hour or two. They not only spike your insulin levels but also assure the post-sugar crash afterward.

- **Fruit juice:** An 8-ounce glass of 100 percent orange juice has 25 grams of sugar. Many other so-called fruit juices are only 10 percent juice, with the rest being high-fructose corn syrup or another sweetener (along with artificial color, artificial flavor, and preservatives).

- **Glazes and sauces:** Kashi Sweet & Sour Chicken entree has 25 grams of sugar. Subway's 6-inch teriyaki chicken sandwich has 17 grams of sugar. When eating out, don't be afraid to request items without sauces.

- **Granola:** Just ⅔ of a cup (a tiny serving!) of organic Cascadian Farm Cinnamon Raisin Granola packs 42 grams of total carbs and 16 grams of sugar.

- **Salad dressing:** Fat-free salad dressings are frequently made mostly of sugar and artificial ingredients. Use organic olive oil and vinegar instead.

Spotting other names for sugar

Not everything that is sugar uses that specific word in the list of ingredients. Here's a reference list of some other names for sugar that you may not recognize:

Agave nectar	Corn syrup
Agave syrup	Corn syrup solids
Barley malt	Crystalized fructose
Beet sugar	Date sugar
Brown rice solids	Dextran
Brown sugar	Dextrose
Buttered syrup	Diastase
Cane juice	Diastatic malt
Cane juice crystals	Evaporated cane juice
Cane sugar	Fructose
Carob syrup	Fruit juice
Confectioners' sugar	Fruit juice concentrate
Corn sugar	Glucose
Corn sweetener	Glucose solids

Golden sugar	Maltose
Golden syrup	Maple syrup
Grape juice concentrate	Molasses
Grape sugar	Raw sugar
High-fructose corn syrup	Refiners' syrup
Honey	Sorghum syrup
Invert sugar	Sucanat
Lactose	Sucrose
Malt	Turbinado sugar
Maltodextrin	

Considering Gluten-Free Eating

Gluten is a plant protein found in wheat, rye, and barley. People trying to reduce their carbohydrate intake often also attempt to reduce gluten consumption because eliminating gluten can potentially eliminate a lot of junk food from the diet. Some people have a confirmed sensitivity or allergy to gluten and cut it out of their diets to avoid the side effects.

Why are so many people sensitive to gluten? These grains are a relatively new addition to the human diet (only about 10,000 years or so), so some scientists theorize that humans haven't yet adapted to digesting this type of food. Enough people exhibit a low-grade allergic reaction to gluten that it — along with dairy, nuts, and GMO soy — has become one of the most common allergens of the day.

Gluten sensitivity doesn't result in anaphylactic shock like some severe food allergies can, but it can cause long-term damage if ignored. Continued consumption of gluten by a gluten-sensitive person can lead to *celiac disease* (sometimes referred to as *celiac sprue*), in which gluten damages the intestines, leading to severe nutrient absorption problems and nutritional deficiencies.

Oats don't contain gluten, but they do contain *peptide sequences* that are very similar to wheat gluten. Oats often cause symptoms in celiac patients similar to wheat, and so I include oats in the list of foods for gluten-sensitive individuals to avoid. In addition, though oats themselves are gluten-free, they can be contaminated with gluten from other grains during distribution and processing (most oats are milled and stored in the same facilities as wheat).

Common symptoms of gluten sensitivity are

- ✔ Bloating, cramping, and flatulence
- ✔ Chronic fatigue

- ✔ Diarrhea or constipation

- ✔ Indigestion

- ✔ Joint pain

- ✔ Mouth sores

- ✔ Skin rashes

- ✔ Ulcers

Humans don't need gluten to stay healthy, so some nutritionists suggest that everyone avoid gluten, even those who aren't exhibiting any symptoms of gluten sensitivity. That doesn't make much sense to me, because avoiding all gluten can be a difficult lifestyle choice, so my suggestion is that you try eating gluten-free only if you fit any of these criteria:

- ✔ You have a confirmed gluten sensitivity.

- ✔ You suffer from an autoimmune disorder like eczema, fibromyalgia, IBS, lupus, or rheumatoid arthritis.

- ✔ You've tried eating gluten-free for a few weeks, and you notice that you feel a lot better if you don't eat it.

If you've been diagnosed with celiac disease or non-celiac gluten sensitivity, removing gluten from your diet is very important. Cheating a little here and there may seem harmless, but it can permanently damage your intestines over time and lead to other serious problems like nutrient malabsorption, osteoporosis, depression, and even intestinal cancer.

Avoiding gluten can be tricky because many common foods have ingredients that may be sources of gluten that aren't obvious. In addition to eliminating wheat, barley, rye, and oats from your diet, be aware that the following foods often contain gluten:

- ✔ Beer and distilled spirits

- ✔ Bouillon cubes

- ✔ Candy (sometimes dusted with wheat flour)

- ✔ Canned soups

- ✔ Cheese spreads or other processed cheese foods (why would you eat this anyway?)

- ✔ Chocolate (sometimes contains malt flavoring from barley)

- ✔ Cold cuts and sausages (may have gluten from cereal fillers)

- ✔ Dip mixes

✔ Dry sauce mixes

✔ Dry-roasted nuts and honey-roasted nuts

✔ French fries or other fried foods in restaurants (often coated with flour)

✔ Gravies — check out thickening agents and liquid base

✔ Instant coffee (a cereal product is sometimes included in the formula)

✔ Lip balms and lipsticks

✔ Many ice creams and frozen yogurt products

✔ Mayonnaise (check ingredients that are used as thickeners)

✔ Precooked hams and turkeys from commercial suppliers (often basted with wheat starch and sugar)

✔ Some toothpastes

✔ Sour cream (may contain modified food starch)

Food labels can list items that contain wheat by other names, such as modified food starch, farina, or bran. If you're gluten-sensitive, you can find more thorough food information on websites like www.gfoverflow.com, www.gluten.net, and www.projectallergy.com. And for a complete overview of life without gluten, check out *Living Gluten-Free For Dummies,* by Danna Korn (Wiley).

Steering Clear of Artificial Sweeteners

As I guide you through your quest to reduce sugar intake, I'd be remiss if I didn't report some research about the long-term health dangers of artificial sweeteners. Much of the available research has been done with animals instead of humans, so I invite you to do your own research and draw your own conclusions.

How chemical sweeteners work

Artificial sweeteners work by causing neuro-excitation in a part of the brain that causes people to perceive a sweet taste. The danger is that these chemical sweeteners overstimulate the neurons to the point where they basically self-destruct. You literally get brain damage from these chemicals!

MSG and NutraSweet are especially dangerous for babies (both in and out of the womb) because infants' brains aren't yet protected by the blood-brain barrier. A possible explanation for the enormous rise of autism in American children is the mothers' use of these chemicals while pregnant (and the prevalence of these chemicals in processed food for babies and toddlers). If you're pregnant or have small children, I encourage you to investigate the research on artificial sweeteners in such journals as the *Journal of Child Neurology, Biomedica Biochimica Acta,* the *International Journal of Neuroscience,* and the *Journal of Neurochemistry.*

Monosodium glutamate (MSG)

Most folks are aware that MSG is bad news. Here's why:

- **Brain damage:** Excessive glutamate in the brain kills glutamate receptors and neurons connected to it. This has huge implications for Alzheimer's and Parkinson's diseases.

- **Hypothalamus damage:** The hypothalamus controls other endocrine glands like the thyroid, adrenal glands, and so on.

- **Increased appetite:** The pro-MSG lobbying website (www.msgfacts.com) used to boast that one of the benefits of MSG for food manufacturers was that it caused people to eat more of their products.

- **Retinal cell damage:** MSG has been proven to cause retinal lesions.

- **Weight gain:** MSG increases the amount of insulin that the pancreas produces and causes leptin resistance. One of the standard laboratory practices to create obese mice and rats is to inject them with MSG. They're even referred to as *monosodium-glutamate-obese rats* in the research reports!

Because MSG gets so much bad publicity, food manufacturers hide it behind these names:

- Hydrolyzed oat flour
- Hydrolyzed vegetable protein
- Malt flavoring
- Natural beef (or chicken) flavoring
- Natural flavoring
- Plant protein extract
- Sodium caseinate
- Spices
- Textured vegetable protein
- Yeast extract

The shameful history of NutraSweet's approval by the FDA

When the FDA was presented with aspartame research in 1980, the doctors on that board unanimously ruled that aspartame should not go on the market. An internal FDA panel concluded the same thing.

When Ronald Reagan took office in 1981, FDA Chairman Gere Goyan was replaced by Dr. Arthur Hayes. Hayes was handpicked by Donald Rumsfeld for this position, and at the time, Rumsfeld was conveniently the CEO of the company that owned the patent on aspartame (G. D. Searle & Company).

But even with the friendly new FDA chairman in place, the agency still rejected aspartame for approval by a three-to-two margin. What reprehensible action did Hayes do next? He added a sixth member to the approval board, one who had promised to vote in favor of aspartame. Then, with a three-to-three tie on the issue, Hayes himself broke the deadlock with his own vote of approval for the introduction of aspartame into the public food supply.

Aspartame (NutraSweet)

Aspartame is an artificial sweetener that was discovered by accident in 1965. Aspartame is composed of two amino acids (aspartic acid and phenylalanine) and is 200 times as sweet as table sugar. Commonly labeled as NutraSweet, it is often found in diet soft drinks, sugar-free chewing gum, and sugar-free mixes like puddings and yogurts. Although it's nearly calorie-free, ingesting large amounts of aspartame may have some dangerous effects:

- **Brain damage:** Like MSG, aspartame kills glutamate receptors and neurons connected to it.

- **Brain tumors:** In experiments to test the safety of aspartame before its approval by the U.S. Food and Drug Administration (FDA), animals that were fed NutraSweet developed 25 times as many brain tumors as the control animals.

- **Increased appetite:** NutraSweet suppresses the production of *serotonin,* one of the neurotransmitters that makes you feel full and satisfied. When your serotonin levels aren't allowed to rise as they normally do when you eat, you crave more and more food.

- **Methanol (wood alcohol):** Aspartame is 10 percent methanol, which, according to the *European Journal of Clinical Nutrition,* "can give rise to formaldehyde, diketopiperazine [a carcinogen], and a number of other highly toxic derivatives."

Sucralose (Splenda)

The good news about sucralose is that it doesn't cross the blood-brain barrier, so it shouldn't cause brain damage. The bad news is that Splenda, the most common sucralose sweetener, is a *chlorocarbon,* which is a known carcinogen (and is used as a pesticide, too). Chlorocarbons have long been known for causing organ, genetic, and reproductive damage.

The FDA approved Splenda as a sweetener in 1998. The approval was based on more than 110 animal and human safety studies. However, out of these 110 studies, only 2 were human studies, consisting of a combined total of 36 people, of which only 23 people actually ingested sucralose. Additionally, the longest of these human trials lasted only *four days* and looked at sucralose in relation to tooth decay, not human toxicity. Sheesh!

The testing of sucralose reveals that it can cause up to 40 percent shrinkage of the *thymus,* a gland that's vital to your immune system.

In animal studies, Splenda reduces the amount of good bacteria in the intestines by 50 percent, acidifies the intestines, and contributes to increases in body weight. It also affects the P-glycoprotein in the body in such a way that certain medications (chemotherapy, AIDS treatment, and drugs for heart conditions) may be rejected by shunting them back into the intestines rather than absorbing them by the body as intended.

What should you do?

Don't eat or drink products with these chemicals (or their hidden pseudonyms) on the label.

Proper nutrition may help protect your brain. The vitamin E and selenium in nuts and seeds and the *anthocyanins* in grapes and berries can play a protective role. There's also good research on the neuroprotective effects of omega-3 fatty acids from fish and supplemental acetyl l-carnitine.

If you must eat or drink something with MSG or NutraSweet, make sure you have some carbohydrates in your system. The damage that these chemicals cause to your brain is much worse when your glucose levels are low. One of the worst things you can do to your brain is drink a diet soda on an empty stomach!

Chapter 4

How Sugar Contributes to Chronic Health Problems

*F*rom a physiology standpoint, processed sugars like table sugar and high-fructose corn syrup are broken down in the digestive system and are dealt with exactly like other carbohydrates from vegetables, fruits, and grains. But the health problems from processed sugars stem from the fact that people get overloaded with far too much sugar, and worse, processed sugars lack the nutrients naturally found in plant carbohydrates — vitamins, minerals, fiber, antioxidants, and protein.

Eating refined sugars loads you up on calories and triggers a gigantic release of insulin, all without adding a single valuable nutrient or a lone gram of fiber or protein. All those empty calories add up, making sugar consumption one of the primary causes of obesity throughout much of the world.

High sugar intake has been proven to lower the effectiveness of your immune system. It also promotes inflammation and produces damaging byproducts. Sugar disrupts the natural energy production of the body's adrenal cortex, so it can lead to chronic fatigue and depression.

So if obesity, diabetes, fatigue, metabolic syndrome, osteoporosis, and inflammatory diseases aren't enough reasons to change your eating habits, perhaps my next book should be *Wheelchairs For Dummies*. You can read about all these health problems — and quite a few more — in this chapter.

Sugar Highs: Looking at Escalating Health Problems

Sugar consumption in the United States has skyrocketed in recent decades, and this increase has resulted in a corresponding rise in obesity, diabetes, and other health problems. The use of high-fructose corn syrup has increased over 1,000 percent (see Figure 4-1) since it first entered the American food supply in 1975!

Notice that consumption of high-fructose corn syrup peaked around the year 2000. The low-fat craze of the 1990s exacerbated the sugar overload in the American food supply. To make fat-free food taste good, manufacturers add a pile of sugar and salt (and often other chemicals that are even worse) to make up for the missing fat. This process exchanges dietary fat for processed sugar and other chemicals, which are harmful.

Figure 4-1:
History of annual consumption of high-fructose corn syrup in the United States.

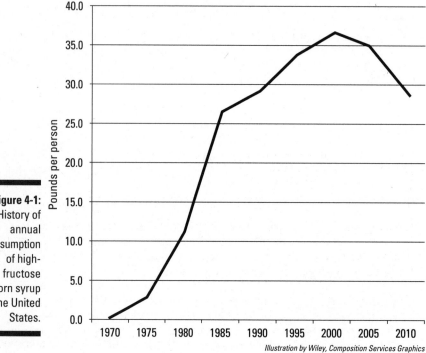

Illustration by Wiley, Composition Services Graphics

The United States leads the world in sugar consumption, and as a result, it also leads the world in diabetes healthcare expenditures. Figure 4-2 shows the costs of diabetes in the United States over the same time period as in Figure 4-1. The American Diabetes Association reports that millions of new cases of diabetes are diagnosed every year in the United States. In addition to the tens of millions of diabetics, 80 million Americans have pre-diabetes (insulin resistance), so unless those people change their eating habits (and I hope you're one who does), there'll be no shortage of diabetes in the years to come. You can read more about diabetes later in this chapter.

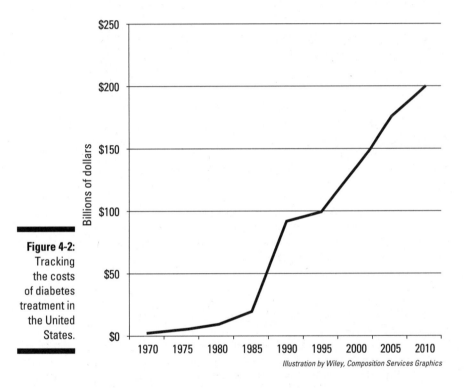

Figure 4-2:
Tracking the costs of diabetes treatment in the United States.

Illustration by Wiley, Composition Services Graphics

Seeing the Psychological Ramifications of Sugar

Sugar is a food, but it has drug-like effects on your brain. Sugar triggers the pleasure center of your brain just like alcohol and cocaine, and it can become just as addictive. Sugar affects the chemistry of both your body and your brain, so sugar addicts commonly struggle with depression, anxiety, or both.

Depression

The primary cause of depression is a problem with the hormone *serotonin,* which is a substance that makes people feel happy and satisfied. Most serotonin is produced in the gut. Many things affect the body's production of serotonin, including attitude, nutrition, and sleep.

Eating sugar and other high-glycemic carbohydrates (carbs that raise your blood sugar quickly; see Chapter 5) like white flour triggers the pancreas to secrete a large dose of insulin to control blood sugar levels (*insulin* is the hormone that shuttles sugar from the blood into cells). Insulin is a precursor to serotonin, so a high insulin level leads to a temporary elevation of serotonin. No wonder they call sugar and carbs *comfort foods!*

Chronic overconsumption of sugar causes the body to produce less serotonin on its own because it starts relying on the external supply from your sugary diet. This lack of natural serotonin production can cause depression and create a situation where you need sugar to feel good, because you're producing less serotonin without it.

To maintain a normal level of endorphins in the brain, the sugar abuser must eat more sugar and carbohydrates to relieve the state of depression and maintain a normal mood level. This causes a vicious cycle of addiction. Interestingly, this is exactly the same cycle that develops with excessive alcohol intake. Alcohol abuse, like sugar abuse, causes many of the endorphin sites to shut down, so to get the feel-good effects normally given by endorphins, the alcoholic must continue to drink alcohol instead.

Additionally, B vitamins (especially folic acid), which are essential for the production of serotonin, are used up to metabolize all that sugar, leaving less for the production of serotonin and other important uses.

Excess *fructose* (a simple sugar I describe in Chapter 3) can exacerbate depression. Research has shown that people who have trouble metabolizing fructose (up to half the population) have lower levels of *tryptophan* (a serotonin precursor). They also have lower serum zinc and folic acid levels, both of which are associated with depression. Women already have lower serum levels of tryptophan than men do (which is likely part of the reason why women are more vulnerable to depression), so depleting tryptophan in the diet with fructose may lead to even lower levels, and thus depression.

Statistically, women are more prone to clinical depression than men for several reasons, one being estrogen. Estrogen activates an enzyme called *hepatic tryptophan 2, 3 dioxygenase* (don't worry; there won't be a quiz) that shifts the metabolism of tryptophan from making serotonin (the happy hormone) to making kynurenic acid (a substance that hinders brain function). Maybe that's why women get "baby brain" or severe mood swings when estrogen levels rise during pregnancy.

Blood sugar spikes actually destabilize the brain through a harmful process called glycation. *Glycation* is the chemical process in the body whereby sugars, proteins, and certain fats become tangled together, making all manner of body tissues stiff and inflexible — including the brain. Glycation causes damage in the body that induces rapid aging effects (see the "Wrinkles" section later in the chapter) and physically shrinks your brain tissue.

According to the Mayo Clinic, people with depression often have low blood levels of the essential fats *eicosapentaenoic acid* (EPA) and *docosahexaenoic acid* (DHA). Good sources of these essential nutrients are cold-water fish like salmon and tuna and distilled fish oil capsules (see Chapter 5 for more information about helpful nutrition supplements). Sugar addicts struggling with depression may want to consider adding extra sources of these important fats to their diet.

Anxiety

Sugar addicts commonly suffer from anxiety. Sugar abuse produces a blood-sugar roller coaster that can trigger anxiety attacks. When blood sugar levels crash, your brain gets desperate for food, and your body can become shaky, weak, confused, and anxious. If you're stressed out all the time, check yourself — do you frequently find yourself breathing shallowly or even unconsciously holding your breath? When is the last time you took a deep breath and dropped your shoulders away from your ears? As blood sugar levels plummet, the brain reacts by sending out a panicked adrenaline alarm, leading to severe anxiety. People who are prone to anxiety attacks generally walk around in a state of heightened stress anyway, so it doesn't take much to push them over the edge — a sugar crash is often just the ticket.

Another way that sugar can cause an anxiety attack is by causing lactic acid to build up in the bloodstream. *Lactic acid* is the final product in the breakdown of blood sugar (glucose) when there's a lack of oxygen. If you're prone to anxiety, a buildup of carbon dioxide and lactic acid in the blood causes a pH change in your brain that signals your amygdala to trigger feelings of anxiety and fear.

Adrenaline junkies often report that they need caffeine or sugar to jump-start their energy in the morning. To calm yourself down and gradually coax your adrenal glands back into normal functioning, start weaning yourself off sugar and coffee, and try green tea instead. Green tea contains less caffeine than coffee and high amounts of the amino acid *l-theanine,* which can help you stay calm and focused. Licorice tea is another smart choice — it's naturally sweet, and it helps improve your adrenal function.

Dealing with Medical Risks and Problems

The estimated annual healthcare costs of obesity, diabetes, depression, cancer, and metabolic syndrome combined are in the hundreds of billions of dollars in the United States alone. That's more than the gross national product of most countries!

Poor nutrition (with sugar abuse leading the way) causes a long list of medical problems, which are mostly preventable through a healthy lifestyle and a high-quality diet. I cover many of these medical problems in the following sections.

Obesity

The Centers for Disease Control and Prevention report that obesity has overtaken cigarette smoking for the number-one spot on the list of healthcare costs.

Overconsumption of sugar causes obesity in two primary ways: excess calories and excess *insulin* (the hormone that shuttles sugar from the blood into cells).

Excess calories

Sugar contains no nutrients to speak of, only calories. Because it lacks fiber and nutrients, sugar bypasses your body's natural *leptin* response (leptin is the hormone that signals your brain that you have enough body fat), so even after eating hundreds of calories in sugar, you don't feel satisfied.

It only takes eating 100 extra calories per day to gain 10 pounds over a year! Sugary junk foods are low in nutrients and high in calories. High-sugar diets cause more sugar cravings and a strong desire for more carbohydrates. Be sure to get your carbohydrates from vegetables, which are high in nutrients and low in calories. The fiber and "crunchy" factor help you feel full. Whole grains are also high in fiber and nutrients.

Fructose (see Chapter 3) appears to affect leptin sensitivity more than other sugars. If you consistently overeat fructose, your brain can become insensitive to leptin — a condition known as *leptin resistance*. Unable to sense leptin, your brain lowers your metabolism to try to conserve fat stores. To replace the missing body fat, your body packages up any dietary fat present in the high-fructose food and stores it as body fat. Common foods with high concentrations of fructose are fruit juice, high-fructose corn syrup, and agave nectar.

Excess insulin

Eating too much sugar at one time leads to a large release of insulin to control the amount of sugar in the bloodstream. High insulin levels erroneously tell the brain that, because the system has excess insulin, your cells must be starving for glucose. In response, your brain creates cravings for carbohydrates and signals your body to store fat. Excess body fat causes insulin resistance, so obesity both *causes* and *is caused by* type 2 diabetes (see the next section for details).

In women, excess insulin also stimulates the ovaries to produce excess testosterone, which can cause infertility by preventing the ovaries from releasing an egg each month. High levels of insulin also increase the conversion of *androgens* (male hormones) to *estrogens* (female hormones), upsetting the delicate balance between the two and having a direct effect on the formation of cystic follicles or cysts in the ovary. For this reason, women with polycystic ovary syndrome (PCOS) must control their insulin levels through diet.

Diabetes

Several types of diabetes exist, but 90 percent of all cases in the United States are *type 2 diabetes,* which is caused by a diet that keeps insulin levels high. Eating too many carbohydrates (especially sugar) leads to excess insulin production and increased body fat. Large amounts of body fat and frequent high insulin levels decrease your ability to respond to your own insulin. This inability of your cells to respond to insulin is termed *insulin resistance,* and it causes your cells to "refuse" the glucose from the blood (for more on this, see the sidebar "Insulin: Comparing normal and impaired function"). When glucose builds up in the blood instead of going into cells, it can lead to serious problems like organ damage, nerve damage (neuropathy), blindness, hearing loss, heart disease, and stroke.

High insulin levels suppress the production of two important hormones: *glucagon* and *growth hormone.* Your body secretes glucagon when your blood sugar levels are low because its job is to trigger the release of fat to be burned for energy. High insulin levels shut down glucagon production, so you can't burn fat.

Your body uses growth hormone for muscle repair and building new muscle tissue. Insulin resistance reduces muscle development, which keeps your metabolism slow.

Insulin: Comparing normal and impaired function

Insulin transports other nutrients besides glucose, including amino acids from protein and lipid molecules from fats. Insulin connects with special *insulin receptors* on cell surfaces and acts as a "key" to open up the cells to receive nutrients. Insulin receptors are on virtually all body tissues, including muscle and fat cells. When you become insulin-resistant, your cells don't respond to insulin properly. This table compares normal insulin response with impaired insulin response:

When insulin receptors function correctly:	**When you have insulin resistance:**
Insulin transports glucose into cells, clearing it from the bloodstream.	Glucose isn't cleared from the bloodstream; the excess sugar damages tissues and creates inflammation.
Glucose is stored in the liver and in muscle cells as *glycogen* for fuel.	Glucose isn't stored properly, and cells get starved for energy. The brain increases cravings for more sugar.
Insulin moves amino acids into muscles, stimulating repair and growth.	Muscles lack essential amino acids and begin to break down.
The insulin/glucagon axis functions properly to break down fat for energy when needed.	Chronically high insulin levels shut off fat burning and stimulate fat storage.

Type 2 diabetes leads to a vicious Catch-22 that makes weight loss more difficult and blood sugar control less reliable. High levels of insulin can send the wrong signals to the brain — by assuming that your cells are starving for glucose, your brain creates cravings for carbohydrates, signals your body to store fat, and orders carbs to be burned for energy rather than body fat.

Type 2 diabetes goes hand in hand with other lifestyle diseases like elevated cholesterol and triglycerides, obesity, and chronic stress issues.

The good news is that you can reverse insulin resistance relatively quickly by lowering your carbohydrate intake and doing some basic exercise (flip to Chapter 12 for advice on exercise).

Cinnamon contains substances (*methylhydroxy chalcone* polymers, if you're a chemistry nerd) that may make insulin receptors more sensitive. Using cinnamon instead of sugar gives you two bonuses in the fight against type 2 diabetes.

Although chronic excess insulin production from a poor diet causes the vast majority of insulin resistance cases, insulin resistance can result from several different problems, including the shape of your insulin (preventing receptor binding), lack of an adequate number of insulin receptors, signaling problems, or glucose transporters not working properly. Whatever the specific cause, the function of insulin becomes impaired, and the same health problems occur. Reducing your carbohydrate intake helps reduce the harmful effects of insulin resistance, regardless of the genesis of your condition.

Liver disease

When you eat fructose, your body sends it to the liver, which converts the fructose molecules into triglycerides (basically fat). The liver exports the triglycerides into the bloodstream, where they're picked up and stored as body fat. The transport system that moves triglycerides from the liver into the bloodstream can only work so fast, so if too much fructose enters the liver at once, the triglycerides accumulate inside the liver, leading to a condition called (unsurprisingly) *fatty liver*.

Due to the enormous amount of high-fructose corn syrup that the average American consumes, nonalcoholic fatty liver disease is now the most common form of liver disease in the United States. In some people with fatty liver disease, the fat that accumulates causes inflammation and scarring of the liver. This more serious form of liver disease is called *nonalcoholic steatohepatitis,* or *NASH* for short. At its most severe, fatty liver disease can progress to liver failure, which means transplant or death.

Sugar and cholesterol

The preceding section on liver disease explains how sugar creates triglycerides. The body makes *very low-density lipoprotein* (VLDL) to transport these extra triglycerides. As the VLDL circulates in the blood, triglycerides are deposited and the particle gets smaller, eventually becoming a *low-density lipoprotein* (LDL), the "bad" cholesterol. The more sugar you eat, the more harmful LDL you're left with.

High insulin levels (from high carbohydrate intake) also raise cholesterol production in the body by stimulating the cholesterol-producing enzyme *HMG-CoA reductase.*

High sugar consumption lowers *high-density lipoprotein* (HDL), the "good" cholesterol that acts as a vacuum cleaner and removes cholesterol from the arterial walls. Low HDL is one of the hallmarks of metabolic syndrome (see the next section). The more sugar you eat, the lower your good HDL and the higher your bad LDL and triglycerides.

Refined sugar contains no fiber, but vegetables, whole grains, and fruits do! Dietary fiber sweeps cholesterol out of the body before it can be absorbed, keeping your arteries clear of buildup that would otherwise turn into dangerous plaque on the arterial walls. Try to eat at least 30 grams of dietary fiber each day.

Metabolic syndrome

Metabolic syndrome (formerly known as *syndrome X*) is a term used to describe the inevitable results of the typical high-sugar diet: abdominal fat, elevated triglycerides, high blood pressure, and high blood sugar levels.

I think metabolic syndrome should be renamed "excess carbohydrate sickness" because that's really what it is. Stop eating so many carbohydrates and your "syndrome" magically disappears!

With a high-carbohydrate diet, the insulin receptors on the cells become less and less sensitive. Because the sugar can no longer enter the cells like it's supposed to, it gets stored as fat instead. Eating a high-sugar diet over time turns your body into a fat-storing factory — you can take in thousands of calories each day, but little of it supplies lean tissue. Your muscle content drops (which lowers your metabolism), while fat storage becomes more and more efficient. All that body fat increases inflammation, and the insulin resistance refuses to let your body think you've had enough food.

The only way to reverse this downward spiral is to drastically reduce your carbohydrate intake and to commit to some short bouts of high-intensity exercise a few times per week (see Chapter 12 for exercise advice).

Figure 4-3 shows the current clinical definition of metabolic syndrome set by the International Diabetes Foundation at the time of this writing.

Hypothyroid disease

According to the American Association of Clinical Endocrinologists, more than 50 million Americans are affected by some type of thyroid disorder. Diet and stress are the two things that most strongly affect your thyroid function.

After you eat too much sugar, you get a large rush of sugar into the bloodstream. This forces your pancreas to release a mountain of insulin that leads to a corresponding low-blood-sugar crash shortly afterward. Low blood sugar not only stimulates more cravings but also triggers a release of the stress hormone *cortisol,* whose job is to break down carbohydrates stored in the muscles to bring blood sugar levels back up to normal. Repeated cortisol releases from episodes of low blood sugar suppress the function of the *pituitary gland,* and without proper pituitary function, your thyroid doesn't function properly.

Central obesity	Waist circumference ≥ 94 centimeters for men, ≥ 80 centimeters for women; there are slightly different values for Asian ethnicities
Plus at least two of the following:	
Elevated triglycerides	≥ 150 milligrams/deciliter, or to be under treatment for elevated triglycerides
Reduced HDL (good) cholesterol	< 40 milligrams/deciliter for men, < 50 milligrams/deciliter for women, or to be under treatment for low HDL cholesterol
Elevated blood pressure	Systolic ≥ 130, diastolic ≥ 85, or to be under treatment for hypertension
Elevated fasting plasma glucose levels	≥ 100 milligrams/deciliter, or previous diagnosis of type 2 diabetes

Figure 4-3:
Defining metabolic syndrome.

Illustration by Wiley, Composition Services Graphics

Low thyroid function and excess sugar form a Catch-22: Low thyroid function slows insulin's clearing of glucose from the blood, and high sugar levels slow thyroid output. When you're *hypothyroid,* your cells aren't very sensitive to glucose, and because your cells don't get the glucose they need, your adrenals release cortisol to increase the amount of glucose available to them. As long as you keep yourself on the sugar-binge-then-crash roller coaster, your thyroid won't work properly.

Another common source of thyroid failure is *Hashimoto's thyroiditis,* an autoimmune condition where the body makes antibodies against its own thyroid tissue. Studies have shown that the insulin spikes caused by high sugar intake increase the destruction of the thyroid gland in people with Hashimoto's disease.

Chronic fatigue

Chronic stress activates the adrenal glands to produce stress hormones like cortisol and epinephrine. Overproduction of these hormones drops your blood sugar because stress hormones make you burn circulating blood sugar for energy instead of body fat. When blood sugar drops, your brain turns on the sugar cravings to replace the burned-off sugar.

When you're stressed out all the time, your adrenal glands can't keep up with the constant workload, so they lose their ability to continue churning out enough hormones to keep glucose in your system. The result is a consistent underproduction of cortisol, which in turn yields low blood sugar, chronic fatigue, and more sugar cravings.

Chronic fatigue doesn't come just from stress; it comes from excess sugar, too. Insulin resistance causes the cells to refuse the action of insulin trying to bring sugar into cells to be burned for energy. The result is more sugar circulating in the bloodstream and less sugar available to be metabolized for energy. This makes you tired — unspeakably tired, no matter how much you sleep. Cells are unable to take up the glucose they require, and muscles can't restock their fuel supplies of glycogen. The whole system begins to shut down and becomes an exhausted, nonfunctional mess.

Fibromyalgia

Fibromyalgia is one of the terms given to the condition of chronic, widespread musculoskeletal pain and fatigue. Emotional stress coupled with inflammation from too much sugar causes the nervous system to remain in an overactive state, keeping muscles "turned on" when they shouldn't be. This causes muscles to go into tight, spastic knots that reduce circulation. As a result of the decrease in blood flow, muscles don't get the oxygen they need, and metabolic waste products start to build up. This activates nerves in the area, causing pain and constant fatigue.

Sugar damages cells through a process called *glycation* that causes muscle tissue and fascia to become stiffer and thicker. This makes chronic pain conditions worse because the inflexible tissue becomes extremely sensitive to touch and movement.

If you have chronic pain, always remember that your body chemistry is affected by your emotions too! Every single thought and emotion you have triggers certain chemical reactions throughout your body. If you truly believe that you're healthy and powerful, your body chemistry moves toward that reality. If you consistently obsess over how bad you feel or you believe that there's always something wrong with you and that you'll never be well, your sickness becomes more deeply rooted in your physiology. Careful what you tell yourself — your brain is listening!

Irritable bowel syndrome

Not surprisingly, your digestive system is one of the first body systems to be affected by your diet. Consistent consumption of fast food, chemicals, and high-sugar food creates a continuous state of inflammation in the gut. High sugar consumption elevates blood acid levels and increases levels of inflammatory markers like *C-reactive protein* and *homocysteine,* and this consistent inflammation can lead to a chronic irritation of the digestive system known as *irritable bowel syndrome* (IBS).

If you're under constant stress, be it emotional stress or physical stress from inflammation, your nervous system stays overstimulated, which results in a decrease in production of digestive enzymes and less movement of the bowels, which makes the irritable bowel condition worse.

If you have a fructose absorption problem (up to half of the population does), the *GLUT5 transporter* in the small intestine doesn't take up fructose as efficiently as it could. That means a lot of undigested fructose travels down to the colon, feeding the bacteria there and leading to bloating, cramping, and diarrhea — all symptoms of irritable bowel syndrome. If you have IBS, avoid consuming too much fructose at one time.

An acidic, high-sugar diet creates an environment in the intestines that kills off the beneficial bacteria (the *intestinal flora*) that colonize the gut. This makes way for harmful organisms to take hold, including parasites, infectious bacteria, and yeast (see the next section). Disrupting the intestinal flora adds to bowel irritation by compromising both digestion and immunity.

Immune system impairment

Research clearly shows that ingesting large amounts of sugar results in a significant decrease in the ability of the immune system to engulf bacteria. This effect occurs rapidly after eating sugar and lasts for several hours afterward. If you eat sugary foods several times per day, you're keeping your immune system in a depressed state almost constantly!

A high-sugar diet destroys the *intestinal flora* — the beneficial bacteria that are crucial to digestion and the immune system's proper functioning. Transitioning to a low-sugar, high-vegetable diet and using a probiotic supplement (see Chapter 5) can help reestablish the intestinal flora and restore your immune system back to normal function. Two common results of faulty immune system function are detailed below.

Yeast infections

Vaginal yeast infections are usually caused by an overgrowth of *Candida albicans,* a fungus normally found in only tiny amounts in dark, damp nooks and crannies of the body. Your immune system usually keeps the amount of *Candida* in check, but when your immune system is compromised, overgrowths aren't uncommon.

Ingesting sugar lowers your immune response almost immediately. A high-sugar diet also reduces the amount of beneficial bacteria in the intestines (as does antibiotic use), further weakening the immune system.

Yeast feeds on sugar, and it grows best in an acidic environment. A high-sugar diet gives it both!

Autoimmune disorders

Your body is under a constant barrage of attacks from not only bacteria and viruses but also pollution, pesticides, radiation, chemicals, carcinogens, metal poisoning, and other exposures both seen and unseen. Your immune system is strongly affected by your diet, your lifestyle, your environment, and your stress level.

One of the theories of the genesis of autoimmune diseases is that, over time, chronic stress and poor diet cause cells to become less efficient at eliminating waste products and toxins. Eventually, these waste products and toxins incorporate themselves into your cell membranes, causing your immune system to identify such cells as being damaged or foreign. At that point, your immune system tags these diseased cells with antibodies and starts attacking them.

High blood-sugar levels damage your body's tissues and trigger an inflammatory response. Chronic inflammation is the hallmark of autoimmune disorders because it keeps the immune system on overdrive.

In addition to causing inflammation, overconsumption of sugar (especially fructose) causes overgrowth of bacteria and yeast in the large intestine, which keeps the immune system on overdrive in an attempt to quell the continuous infestation.

Bone loss

Excess sugar has a negative effect on all your tissues, including your bones and teeth. This section explains how sugar contributes to problems with bone density and tooth decay.

Osteoporosis and osteopenia

Osteoporosis (and its precursor, *osteopenia*) are conditions that describe varying degrees of bone loss (also referred to as *thinning of the bones*). Bone loss occurs when your body breaks down bone tissue faster than it makes new bone. When your bones are too thin, you're at risk of dangerous and debilitating fractures — one in five hip fracture patients dies within a year of their injury! Without getting too technical, sugar contributes to osteoporosis by raising the acidity of the blood, requiring your body to restore its acid/alkaline balance by breaking down bone tissue to flood the blood with calcium to neutralize the excess acid.

After overdosing on sugar, the resulting sugar crash causes a significant increase in your cortisol levels. Long-term elevation of cortisol can cause severe bone loss.

Diets high in grains can promote bone density problems too, because the *phytic acid* in grains binds to calcium and other minerals, limiting absorption. For strong bones, eat your veggies, decrease the bread, and stay away from the sweets!

Tooth decay and bad breath

Tooth decay starts when you eat sugar, and bacteria metabolize the carbohydrates to form acids that dissolve tooth enamel. Bacteria multiply rapidly in the wet, sugary environment of the addict's mouth, and a decayed tooth soon results.

Research shows that frequent consumption of sugar, particularly when eaten alone between meals, promotes tooth decay. Sugars and starches are less cavity-producing when ingested along with protein, fat, and water. So if you want to keep your teeth healthy, don't snack on sugar.

The bacteria that live off the sugar stuck to your tooth enamel produce smelly byproducts that can give you bad breath. These bacteria can cause infection and inflammation of the gums, too.

Wrinkles

Sugar causes *glycation* of tissues in the body, making them stiffer and less elastic. Sugar in your system attaches to proteins to form harmful new molecules called *advanced glycation end products* (or, appropriately, AGEs for short). The more sugar you eat, the more AGEs you develop.

Glycated tissue yields rapid aging effects, including loss of elasticity of the skin (wrinkles) and cataracts. AGEs deactivate your body's natural antioxidant enzymes, leaving your skin more vulnerable to sun damage.

In addition to cutting back on the amount of sugar you eat, look for skin products that contain compounds like *aminoguanidine* and *carcinine,* which have been shown to block the formation of AGEs.

Part II

Developing Your Low-Sugar or No-Sugar Food Plan

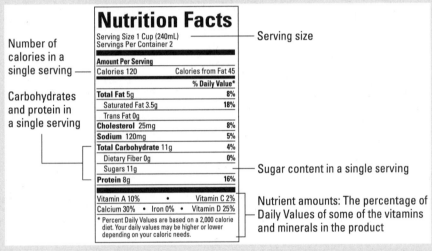

| Number of calories in a single serving | **Nutrition Facts** | Serving size |
| Carbohydrates and protein in a single serving | Serving Size 1 Cup (240mL)
Servings Per Container 2 | |

Nutrition Facts

Serving Size 1 Cup (240mL)
Servings Per Container 2

Amount Per Serving

Calories 120   Calories from Fat 45

% Daily Value*

Total Fat 5g   8%

Saturated Fat 3.5g   18%

Trans Fat 0g

Cholesterol 25mg   8%

Sodium 120mg   5%

Total Carbohydrate 11g   4%

Dietary Fiber 0g   0%

Sugars 11g

Protein 8g   16%

Vitamin A 10%   •   Vitamin C 2%

Calcium 30%   •   Iron 0%   •   Vitamin D 25%

* Percent Daily Values are based on a 2,000 calorie diet. Your daily values may be higher or lower depending on your caloric needs.

- Number of calories in a single serving
- Carbohydrates and protein in a single serving
- Serving size
- Sugar content in a single serving
- Nutrient amounts: The percentage of Daily Values of some of the vitamins and minerals in the product

Illustration by Wiley, Composition Services Graphics

web extras

Find out why a high-sugar diet makes losing weight so hard at www.dummies.com/extras/beatingsugaraddiction.

In this part . . .

- ✔ Create a foundation of good nutrition in order to better manage your appetite and stay craving-free.

- ✔ Take charge of managing your calories and practicing portion control.

- ✔ Consider adding nutrition supplements to your daily routine for health and nutrition help.

- ✔ Tap into the benefits of a sugar detox and navigate traditional and alternative methods for dealing with sugar abuse.

Chapter 5

Creating a Sustainable Plan: The Basics of Nutrition and Portions

In This Chapter

▶ Getting enough (and the right kind of) protein, carbs, fats, and water

▶ Choosing natural produce, meat, dairy, eggs, and fish

▶ Watching your calories and portions

▶ Fortifying your diet with the right nutrition supplements

*T*he avalanche of nutrition advice available from the media and the Internet can be overwhelming. My goal for this chapter is to deliver the facts to you as they are currently understood — without gimmicks or special "diets" — and give you a system for designing a sensible, sustainable, low-sugar eating plan that works for you from this day forward.

This chapter talks about the basic *macronutrients* (protein, carbohydrates, and fat) that you need to build your nutritional foundation, as well as the importance of water. I also discuss calories and portion control and deliver an important explanation of why a calorie is not just a calorie.

Another topic of discussion is nutrition supplements for improving overall health and for reducing sugar cravings, too!

Creating a Sugar-Free Foundation with the Big Four

Even though the focus of this book is freeing yourself from the unhealthy grip of sugar, I invite you to think on a larger scale and create a new, healthy nutrition system for yourself (and for your family, if you're feeding them too).

A nutrition foundation starts with the three *macronutrients* (protein, carbohydrates, and fats) and water. These are the big four that you can't live without.

The macronutrients are the components of foods that supply you with calories to stay alive and with raw materials to maintain and renew your cells, muscles, organs, brain, and all the other tissues.

Picking protein

Dietary protein is essential for maintaining the structure of your body. All the soft tissues in the body — muscles, ligaments, tendons, organs, and even skin and hair — are made of protein. Most enzymes are proteins, and your body uses proteins to catalyze almost all the reactions in living cells, so proteins control virtually every cellular process. The major neurotransmitters are proteins, and your immune cells and antibodies all have proteins attached to them. Protein is ubiquitous in the body and thus is a fundamental part of human dietary requirements.

Most of the high-quality sources of protein are sugar-free, but be advised that dairy sources of protein are often higher in carbohydrates than meat, poultry, fish, and eggs. Some protein is present in grains and legumes too.

You digest protein more slowly than carbohydrates, so it slows blood sugar release and helps you feel satisfied for a longer period of time. Eating protein also boosts your metabolic rate more than eating fat or carbohydrates.

Understanding protein quality

So why are some proteins better than others? What makes a good protein? Proteins are made up of strings of *amino acids.* Nutrition scientists have identified 22 specific amino acids that are found in the human body. These amino acids combine in different ways to synthesize proteins that the body uses for building structures and for various chemical and enzymatic processes.

Your body is very good at being able to rig stuff and pull off stunts to obtain adequate nutrients and stay alive. One of these cool skills is that your body can actually manufacture many of these 22 amino acids if it's supplied with 9 specific amino acids. These 9 amino acids are termed *essential amino acids* because the body can't manufacture them — they must be obtained through food. One of the criteria used to determine the quality of a protein is its content of essential amino acids.

If your food doesn't supply enough of even one of the essential amino acids, your body will begin to break down its protein structures — muscle and organs — to obtain the missing amino acids. The human body doesn't store excess amino acids for later use, like it does with fat and carbohydrate. Amino acids must be present in the food, so it's important to try to eat a quality protein source every few hours throughout the day to avoid muscle tissue breakdown. This breakdown, by the way, is called *catabolism,* and it results in lowered metabolism and less fat-burning potential.

Finding sources of protein

The best protein sources come from animals in the form of meat, poultry, eggs, fish, and dairy. Plants like soy, nuts, and legumes can also supply you with some dietary protein. Following is a summary of these protein sources, in descending order of *biological value* (protein quality).

The healthiest foods come from organic, natural sources. That means you'll ideally use pasture-fed, hormone-free meat, poultry, and eggs and wild-caught fish and shrimp (not farmed) whenever possible. Choose organic vegetable proteins to steer clear of pesticides and genetically modified food. See the later section "Eating Natural Foods" for details.

Getting protein from animal sources

All proteins from animal sources are complete proteins, meaning that they contain all the essential amino acids you need for creating structural and functional proteins. You can get protein from the following sources (the highest-quality sources are at the top of the list):

- **Whey:** Powdered whey protein, which is derived from dairy but is lactose-free, scores highest in all the protein efficiency ratings and tops the list as the highest-quality protein per calorie. (I cover whey protein later, in the "Adding Supplements for Health and Help" section.)

- **Eggs:** Eggs provide protein and healthy fat, along with vitamins and *carotenoids* that can reduce your risk of developing cataracts and age-related macular degeneration. Eggs also contain *choline,* a nutrient that's essential to normal cell structure and proper signaling of nerve cells. The egg white contains most of the protein, and the yolks provide the other healthy nutrients.

- **Fish:** Fresh, wild-caught fish is a good source of protein, B-vitamins, selenium, and omega-3 fats.

- **Lean meats:** When choosing beef, pork, or lamb, buy from local farmers who raise grass-fed, hormone-free livestock. Bison and venison are other popular meats that are relatively low in fat, and they're typically free from antibiotics and hormones.

- **Poultry:** Don't get stuck in a boring chicken or turkey rut — duck, ostrich, goose, quail, and Cornish hens are all yummy, too!

- **Dairy:** Milk, cottage cheese, and Greek yogurt can be decent sources of protein, although the carbohydrate content of many dairy products starts to get high. Cheese is mostly fat, so it's not a great protein source unless it's low-fat or nonfat. You can also experiment with other, more exotic dairy proteins, like goat's milk or kefir if you're feeling adventurous. One strong bonus to dairy products is the high calcium content.

Getting protein from plants

Soy is a complete protein, so soybeans (and edamame, which is just a soybean picked before it's ripe), soy milk, tofu, and powdered soy protein are at the top of the list for quality vegetable proteins. Soy reliably lowers cholesterol and triglycerides, and there's good evidence that the *isoflavones* in soy can help prevent breast cancer.

Most plant sources of proteins — beans, nuts, peas, and lentils — are generally lacking in one or more essential amino acids. Because of this, you need to combine different plant proteins every day to provide a complete spectrum of the essential amino acids. One bonus of plant protein is that it's an excellent source of fiber and phytonutrients that you can't get from animal proteins.

Grains combined with legumes form complete proteins, as do legumes with seeds/nuts. Although dairy foods are complete proteins, they contain extra amino acids to complete the missing profile in grains, so I include some grains-and-dairy combinations in the following list of plant combinations that make complete proteins:

- ✔ **Grains with legumes:** Rice and beans, pea or bean soup and whole-grain crackers, peanut butter on whole-grain bread, pasta fagioli (pasta and beans), hummus and pita bread, pinto beans and corn bread, couscous and black beans, lentil curry and rice, tortillas and refried beans, lentils and bulgur

- ✔ **Grains with dairy:** Cereal and milk, oatmeal and milk, granola and yogurt, macaroni and (real) cheese, grilled cheese sandwich, cheese tortellini

- ✔ **Legumes with seeds/nuts:** Mixed green salad with kidney beans and slivered almonds and sunflower seeds, lentil soup with walnut loaf, chickpea trail mix with nuts and seeds, tahini with peanuts

Consuming carbohydrates

Carbohydrates are the body's primary fuel source. You need carbohydrates in your diet to provide energy to each cell, to feed your brain, and to fuel your muscles and organs. If you don't eat enough carbohydrates, your body will break down muscle tissue to make some!

Are carbs good or bad?

Despite their importance, carbs have become the big bad wolf in the world of weight loss and health consciousness. Some of this thinking is justified because all carbs are definitely not created equal, but categorizing carbohydrates as purely good or purely bad is inaccurate. The physiological response that you get from eating carbohydrates depends on the type, the amount, what else you eat with them, and the current state of your body's chemistry — carbs are definitely not black or white!

Dietary carbohydrates are found in these foods:

- ✔ Grain products like pastas, breads, and cereals

✔ Some milk products like yogurt and milk (other dairy foods like cheese and cottage cheese are very low in carbohydrates)

✔ Sugars like table sugar, syrup, sweetened beverages, honey, and sweets

✔ Vegetables, fruits, and legumes

That's right, vegetables are carb sources. I counsel hundreds of people every year, and many of them are surprised to hear that. Generally, when people tell me they've "cut out carbs," they usually mean they've stopped eating wheat and sugar. That's fine — you don't have to eat wheat or sugar to be healthy. But if you really cut out all carbohydrates, you'd be in metabolic trouble pretty quickly.

You evaluate a carbohydrate in two important ways. The first (and most important) is to consider its overall content of nutrients, fiber, and calories. You should aim for eating mostly vegetables (and some fruit) because they're loaded with nutrients and fiber and are generally very low in calories. Carbohydrates from processed grains and sugary foods are generally high in calories and low in fiber and nutrients. The second is glycemic load, which I discuss next.

Understanding glycemic load

Besides overall nutritional value, the second consideration of a carbohydrate's value is determining how fast it breaks down in digestion and how much sugar enters the bloodstream. Carbohydrate foods differ in how much sugar (and calories) they contain in a given volume of food and also in the speed at which they're broken down into glucose. The amount of sugar and its breakdown speed are combined into a rating system known as the *glycemic load.* The lower the glycemic load, the less the food affects your blood sugar (compare Figures 5-1 and 5-2).

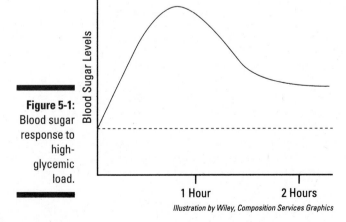

Figure 5-1:
Blood sugar response to high-glycemic load.

Illustration by Wiley, Composition Services Graphics

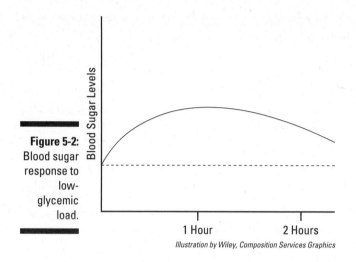

Figure 5-2:
Blood sugar
response to
low-
glycemic
load.

Illustration by Wiley, Composition Services Graphics

Table 5-1 shows some common foods and their glycemic loads for one serving (see the section "Portion distortion: Understanding how much is too much" later in the chapter for help with serving sizes). The lower a food's glycemic load, the less it affects your blood sugar and insulin levels.

As a rule of thumb, most nutrition experts consider glycemic loads less than 10 to be low and glycemic loads more than 20 to be high. Sticking to foods with a low glycemic load is important for diabetics, but even if you're not diabetic, aiming for low-glycemic foods (thus keeping insulin levels lower) can help you lose weight, especially when you eat protein and/or fat with carbohydrates.

Table 5-1   Glycemic Loads of One Serving of Common Foods

Low Glycemic Load	Medium Glycemic Load	High Glycemic Load
Apple: 6	Banana: 12	Apple juice, unsweetened: 30
Beans (average): 6–10	Bread, sourdough: 15	Bagel, white: 24
Beets: 5	Buckwheat: 16	Baguette with butter and strawberry jam: 26
Bran cereal: 8	Cereal, whole-grain: 16	Baked potato, russet: 26
Cantaloupe: 4	Honey: 12	Cake with frosting: 20
Carrots: 2	Muffin, banana oat: 17	Cereal, cornflakes: 21
Chickpeas: 8	New potatoes: 12	Corn, sweet: 20

Low Glycemic Load	Medium Glycemic Load	High Glycemic Load
Grapes: 8	Oatmeal, slow cook: 14	Oatmeal, instant: 30
Milk, skim: 4	Orange juice: 12	Pancakes, buckwheat, gluten-free: 23
Orange: 5	Pretzels: 16	Pasta, boiled: 23
Peach: 5	Rice, wild: 18	Raisins: 28
Peanuts: 1		Rice milk: 29
Peas: 4		Rice, white: 43
Pineapple: 7		Soda, sugared: 23
Popcorn: 8		
Soybeans: 1		
Strawberries: 1		
Whole-wheat bread: 10		

When counseling new clients, every day I hear statements like, "I heard bananas were bad for you," or, "I thought I wasn't supposed to eat potatoes." You must understand that glycemic load by itself doesn't make a food good or bad. It's just a ballpark indication of how a particular food may affect your insulin levels. Combining carbs with protein and fat (which you should do) reduces your insulin response to the carbohydrates and therefore lowers the glycemic load of the entire meal.

Be careful not to base your food choices solely on carbohydrate content or glycemic load. When you look at only one aspect of food, you overlook other important considerations like fiber, vitamins and minerals, dietary fat, and total calories. Many foods with higher glycemic loads are very nutritious, and some low-glycemic foods (like potato chips) aren't very good choices!

If you'd like to read about carbohydrates in more detail, Chapter 3 talks about complex carbs versus simple carbs, enriched grains versus whole grains, fiber content, and insulin control. If you really want to dive into details with the glycemic load concept, read Meri Raffetto's excellent *The Glycemic Index Diet For Dummies* (Wiley).

Choosing the right fats

Dietary fat has been bedeviled in the past as the primary contributor to obesity and heart disease. As nutrition science progresses, it has become clear that dietary fat is a very important component of nutrition. Your body uses fats to produce hormones, transmit nerve impulses, regulate the immune system, and create cell membranes. Fat provides taste to foods and helps you feel full. Fat takes a long time to digest, so it slows the release of sugar into the bloodstream.

Fat is the most efficient source of food energy; each gram of dietary fat provides approximately nine calories of energy for the body, compared with about four calories per gram from carbohydrate or protein.

Vitamins A, D, E, and K are fat-soluble, meaning they can only be digested, absorbed, and transported in conjunction with fats.

Avoiding bad fats

Different types of dietary fat have different effects on the body. Two types of potentially harmful dietary fat are

- **Saturated fat:** This type of fat comes mainly from animal sources of food. Saturated fat from animals that are fed an inflammatory diet (GMO grain and corn instead of grass, perpetual antibiotics, growth hormones, and so on) can raise your inflammatory markers, which increases your risk of cardiovascular disease and other health problems.

- **Trans fat:** Trans fats are created when unsaturated fats (like oils) are heated too much, such as when food is deep-fried. Trans fats are also intentionally added to processed food by a process called *hydrogenation.* This process creates artificial fats that don't spoil as fast as naturally occurring oils, but these Frankenstein fats are toxic to the body.

   Some of the health problems associated with trans fat consumption are increased inflammation, increased cholesterol and triglyceride levels, disruption of the metabolism of essential fats, and increased risk of diabetes.

Fortunately, food manufacturers in the United States must now list the trans fat content of their products on the nutrition facts label, and many companies are actively attempting to remove trans fats from their manufacturing process.

Here are some tips for minimizing trans fats in your diet:

- Avoid eating fried foods and commercially baked goods.
- Don't eat foods with "hydrogenated" in the ingredients.
- Try not to overheat any oil that you cook with.

Seeking out good fats

Not all dietary fat is harmful! You want to consume adequate amounts of healthy fats in your diet. Here are some suggestions for foods high in healthy, unsaturated fats:

- ✔ Avocado
- ✔ Fatty fish (salmon, tuna, mackerel, anchovy)
- ✔ Nuts
- ✔ Oils (olive oil, canola oil, borage oil, grapeseed oil)

Of particular importance are types of unsaturated fats called *omega-3* fatty acids, found primarily in fish, nuts, and some oils. These have a number of heart-healthy effects, including reducing triglyceride levels, raising HDL ("good") cholesterol, "thinning" the blood, reducing levels of homocysteine, and lowering blood pressure.

Two essential omega-3 fatty acids are found primarily in fish: *EPA (eicosapentaenoic acid)* and *DHA (docosahexaenoic acid)*. Research shows that EPA and DHA serve as powerful natural anti-inflammatory agents, lessen the effects of depression, and protect the cardiovascular system. These fats are particularly important to the function of the brain and nervous system.

Technically, the body can manufacture both EPA and DHA from another essential fatty acid — *alpha-linolenic acid* (ALA), found in flaxseed oil, canola oil, soy oil, and walnut oil. However, this conversion is very inefficient (less than 10 percent), so it's virtually impossible to convert enough ALA into adequate amounts of essential fats. Fish oil (or krill oil, if you're not allergic to shellfish) supplementation seems to be the best option (see the later section "Fish oil for essential fats" for details on supplements).

Drinking water: A vital key to craving control

The human body is mostly water. Without it, people would have no cells, no nerve impulses, and no metabolic processes. Even a small amount of dehydration (2 to 3 percent) can result in fatigue, low blood pressure, elevated heart rate, headaches, dry skin, constipation, and decreased mental function.

The part of your brain that controls the thirst sensation is called the *hypothalamus.* Guess what else the hypothalamus controls? Hunger! When you're dehydrated, the hypothalamus kicks in and triggers thirst. This can also trigger food cravings, as you've probably experienced.

Healthy eating at a glance

What you eat is the biggest determinant of your health, so make smart, healthy choices. Your body deserves it! Here are the basics of a healthy, sugar-free eating plan:

1. Eat sensible portions of nutrient-rich foods every three to four hours:

 ✔ Healthy fats — fish oil, nuts, olive oil

 ✔ Healthy protein — whey, wild-caught fish, eggs and meat from pasture-fed animals, non-GMO soy

 ✔ Lots of plants (low-sugar carbohydrates) — dark and brightly colored vegetables, fruits, legumes, and whole grains are generally considered to be the most nutrient-rich plant foods

2. Minimize consumption of highly processed foods.

3. At every meal, eat a *protein* and a *plant.* Don't eat too much at one time.

4. Eat breakfast every day.

5. Drink at least 64 ounces of distilled water throughout the day.

6. Don't eat too much food at night — eat to fuel what you plan to do for the next four hours.

Drinking enough water is one of the easiest ways to keep cravings in check. Doing so also cuts down on your desire for other, less-healthy beverages. Downing a cold glass of water is one of the first things you should do when a sugar craving strikes (see Chapter 9).

 Current recommendations for water intake range from a minimum of 64 ounces daily (eight glasses) to a maximum of one ounce per pound of body weight. Try this — pour distilled water into four pint-sized (16 ounces) stainless-steel water bottles and see how much of it you drink on an average day. (See the later section "Drinking clean water" for info on why I recommend distilled water.)

Eating Natural Foods

Your body is designed to run on natural foods like vegetables, meat, eggs, fruit, fish, nuts, and seeds. When you start to stray from that nutrition foundation by eating lots of processed foods, you lose vital nutrients and consume large amounts of manmade chemicals. To make convenience or packaged foods, companies add chemicals like artificial flavors, chemical coloring, preservatives, emulsifiers, hydrogenated oils, and high-fructose corn syrup and other cheap sweeteners to extend shelf life and add "taste." Sticking with natural foods instead of processed foods delivers more nutrition and less sugar, preservatives, artificial flavors and colors, and other chemicals.

In this section I explain the difference between organic and conventional produce and fill you in on the important differences between food that comes from pasture-fed, antibiotic-free animals and food from industrial feedlot operations.

Picking produce

Sixty or seventy years ago, farmers used crop rotation and manure to keep their soil healthy. Today, the industrial agriculture business uses chemical fertilizers in the ground and covers genetically modified plants with pesticides and herbicides. After harvest, the companies treat the produce with additional chemicals to delay ripening and spoilage while the food is shipped halfway across the world! The nutrition content of this produce is severely compromised. Buying organic produce from local farmers (or growing your own!) ensures that you get the freshest, most nutritious food available, without all the added chemicals. You also get produce that's picked at its peak ripeness, making it more appealing to eat!

If organic produce stresses your grocery budget, flip to Chapter 6 for advice on organic versus conventional produce. Eating whole foods like vegetables, fruits, and nuts is important for vitamins, minerals, fiber, and phytonutrients, whether they're organic or not!

You should seek out vegetables that aren't genetically modified — *Non-GMO* is the term to look for. Because no one knows the long-term health consequences of engineered food, GMO food has been banned in all of Europe (and in dozens of non-European countries, too). You can download the "Non-GMO Shopping Guide" from www.BeatingSugarAddiction.com.

Buying meat, dairy, eggs, and fish

Animals in commercial feedlot facilities are fed unnatural foods loaded with hormones and antibiotics so that the animals fatten quicker and can survive the diseases that crowded, infected living conditions produce. Eating these types of animal products increases inflammation in your body and raises your risk of heart disease and cancer.

Here are some tips for choosing healthier animal products:

✔ **Fish and seafood:** Wild-caught seafood is a great source of protein and essential fats. Sadly, the oceans have become contaminated with mercury, polychlorinated biphenyls (PCBs), and other poisons, so nowadays you must limit the amount of fish in your weekly diet. This is especially important for pregnant women and young children. Visit http:// water.epa.gov for current recommendations on contaminated fish and shellfish consumption.

✔ **Meat and dairy:** Organic, free-range livestock (and the dairy foods from them) have a better nutrition profile — more healthy fats and nutrients and less inflammatory chemicals — than food from commercial feedlot animals, so buy your food from local organic farms.

✔ **Poultry and eggs:** Aim to buy chicken and turkey meat raised without antibiotics and growth hormones in their feed. Whenever possible, choose eggs from pasture-fed chickens, which have less cholesterol and more vitamins and omega-3s (and the living conditions for chickens in industrial operations are atrocious).

Drinking clean water

My recommendation is to drink distilled water. Water filters remove some of the large contaminants and bacteria, but distilling water is the only way to remove all the mercury, lead, pesticides, pharmaceutical residue, PCBs, live-stock runoff, and other hazards that seep into the groundwater. Get your minerals from food and from a high-quality supplement, and don't worry about the tiny amount that's missing from distilled water.

Managing Calories and Portion Control

In nutrition, a *calorie* is the measure of the amount of energy contained in a food. Your body breaks down foods (burns calories) to provide energy to move, think, and keep all the metabolic processes going. The three macro-nutrients (protein, fat, and carbohydrate) have calories. Protein contains approximately four calories per gram, as does carbohydrate. Fat has nine calories per gram, and alcohol has seven.

In this section, you explore the quality of calories, find out how many calories you need, and look at what size your portions should be.

Realizing that a calorie isn't just a calorie

One of the common nutrition mantras that continues to spew from pop medical publications is that the only thing that determines weight loss or weight gain is calories in versus calories out. This is just not true — what happens to the calories you eat is highly dependent on what kind of calories they are and also on the physiological state of the eater.

Let's take two subjects as examples: Woman A splits up 1,200 calories of vegetables and lean protein into five meals every day. Woman B doesn't eat during the day and then gobbles 1,200 calories' worth of donuts every night before bed. These two women will have very different bodies and health profiles, even though they both eat the same number of calories every day. A calorie is *not* just a calorie!

To stay healthy and lean, be sure to take in most of your calories from high-nutrient foods, not *empty calories* (calories without nutrition value).

Determining how many calories you need

If you eat more calories than you need, your body stores the excess as fat. Sugar is a particularly troublesome source of calories because it's often very low in nutrients and it triggers cravings for even more.

A pound of body fat has 3,500 calories, so to lose 1 pound, you need to "release" 3,500 calories. Eating just 100 fewer calories every day yields a loss of 10 pounds in a year. Conversely, if you overeat 100 calories every day, you'll gain 10 pounds in a year!

Individual calorie requirements vary greatly depending on personal metabolism and activity levels, but you can get a decent ballpark number from one of these methods:

- ✔ **The Harris-Benedict formulas:** Nutritionists have used these two formulas for a long time because they give a reasonable approximation of a person's caloric needs:

  Men = 66 + (6.23 × weight in pounds) + (12.7 × height in inches) − (6.8 × age)

  Women = 665 + (4.35 × weight in pounds) + (4.7 × height in inches) − (4.7 × age)

- ✔ **Calorie approximation by activity:** This method of estimating calorie requirements takes your activity into account. Multiply your weight in pounds by one of these activity modifiers:

  × 10 if you're sedentary

  × 13 if you're moderately active (exercise three days per week for at least 30 minutes)

  × 15 if you're very active (exercise for more than five hours per week)

You'll probably find that if you stick to low-glycemic foods (vegetables, lean proteins, and healthy fats), you'll start losing weight without having to worry about tracking calories!

A balanced diet: Finding the right ratios

For years, Americans have been duped into believing that a grain-based, low-fat diet is the best way to combat obesity. As the consistent and appalling rise in obesity and diabetes continues, it's clear that a new set of nutrition guidelines is in order.

Fortunately, the new set of U.S. Department of Agriculture recommendations for the proper ratio of food groups (from www.choosemyplate.gov) is a considerable improvement from the old food pyramid shown in Figure 5-3, which had as its foundation 6 to 11 servings of grains. MyPlate, shown in Figure 5-4, currently recommends that half your plate be filled with vegetables and fruits, one quarter with protein, and one quarter with grains, along with a serving of dairy. The new guidelines are reasonable but still not ideal.

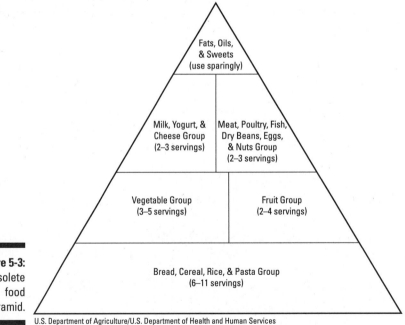

Figure 5-3:
Obsolete
food
pyramid.

U.S. Department of Agriculture/U.S. Department of Health and Human Services

Illustration by Wiley, Composition Services Graphics

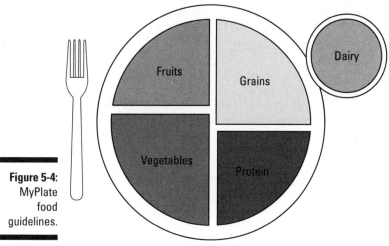

Figure 5-4:
MyPlate
food
guidelines.

Illustration by Wiley, Composition Services Graphics

By combining current available research and 20 years of experience in nutrition counseling, I've determined that most individuals with average calorie expenditure — which, in the United States, means somewhere between completely sedentary and moderately active — function best with approximately equal ratios of calories from protein, fat, and carbohydrate in the diet, creating the 30/30/40 plate shown in Figure 5-5.

If you can eat 30 percent of your calories from protein, 30 percent from healthy fats, and 40 percent from carbohydrates (mostly vegetables), you can stay lean, healthy, and craving-free! This type of insulin-controlled eating is especially important for those with diabetes.

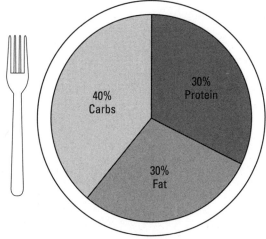

Figure 5-5:
The 30/30/40
plate.

Illustration by Wiley, Composition Services Graphics

Portion distortion: Understanding how much is too much

Increased calorie consumption is one of the three primary causes of obesity in Americans (along with increased sugar consumption and lack of physical activity). Portions and calorie content have risen consistently over the decades, and Americans have the waistlines to prove it!

Here are some comparisons of portion sizes in the 1980s versus today:

Portions and Calories in the 1980s	*Portions and Calories Today*
8 ounce coffee with milk and sugar: 90 calories	Frappuccino: 16 ounces, 350–500 calories
Blueberry muffin: 1.5 ounces, 210 calories	Blueberry muffin: 5 ounces, 500 calories
Chicken stir-fry: 2 cups, 435 calories	Chicken stir-fry: 4 cups, 850 calories
Bagel: 3 inch diameter, 140 calories	Bagel: 5–6 inches diameter, 350 calories

To become accustomed to what a normal serving size is, put out your usual portion of food, measure it, and then compare your serving size to what's on the nutrition label. You may be surprised (or maybe horrified?) to find that your "normal" portion of pasta or breakfast cereal is actually three or four servings!

To become more skilled at eyeballing portions, refer to this handy list until judging your portion sizes becomes second nature:

- ✔ Baseball or computer mouse = a serving of starch like pasta, potatoes, or rice
- ✔ Compact disc = a serving of bread
- ✔ Deck of cards = a serving of meat or fish
- ✔ Golf ball = ¼ cup, a serving of nuts
- ✔ Half your thumb (knuckle to tip) = 1 teaspoon
- ✔ Tennis ball = ½ cup
- ✔ Your fist = a serving of fruit

Adding Supplements for Health and Help

Fortifying your diet with the right nutrition supplements can help fend off sugar cravings and add a much-needed boost to your health and vitality. Proper supplementation is an important component of long-term health and wellness because it's difficult to obtain all the vitamins, minerals, essential fats, and phytonutrients that you need to defend against the onslaught of dangerous chemicals found in the food supply and the environment.

These days your body simply has more to deal with — more stress, more chemicals, more radiation, and more pollutants. To stay healthy, you need serious help, including stress management, smart choices in food, and extra nutrition support.

In addition to choosing nutritious, chemical-free foods (see the earlier section "Eating Natural Foods" for details), you may want to consider the nutrition supplements explained in the next few sections.

These nutrition supplements may not be appropriate for every individual. Some nutrients can cause problems in people with certain medical conditions or can interact with particular medications. You should consult a qualified practitioner for advice concerning your individual situation.

Multivitamin/mineral supplement with B-complex

Chemical fertilizers have depleted the mineral content of the soil used in farming. Organic farming has begun a positive turnaround, but it will take decades for the soil to recover. To ensure that your body has the necessary amounts of the missing minerals — nutrients like chromium, selenium, magnesium, and copper that are no longer in the soil — you can use a basic multivitamin/mineral supplement for nutritional insurance. Remember that deficiencies in nutrients can trigger cravings!

The B-vitamins are critical for energy production, dopamine production, and brain function. B vitamins have been shown to lower the risk of diabetes and to decrease the incidence of migraines. If your multivitamin/mineral supplement doesn't contain high doses of B vitamins, you can take an additional B-complex separately.

Recommended brands of quality multivitamin/mineral supplements are available at www.BeatingSugarAddiction.com.

Vitamin C, an immune booster

Infections and stress eat up vitamin C. Supplemental vitamin C boosts your immunity by improving components of the immune system that have cool-sounding names like *natural killer cells* and *lymphocytes.* Vitamin C helps maintain the integrity of cells and helps protect them against oxidative damage. Vitamin C is also important for iron absorption, wound healing, and maintaining the strength of blood capillaries.

Recommended dosage of supplemental vitamin C is 500 to 2000 milligrams per day. Use vitamin C with *rose hips* or *acerola cherry* because the antioxidant benefits of vitamin C are magnified when you combine it with flavonoids and other compounds in these plants.

An interesting fact: Humans are one of the few mammals that can't make their own vitamin C. The others are apes, guinea pigs, and fruit bats.

If you're new to vitamin C supplements, use a small dose for a few days, and gradually build up your dose over the course of a few weeks. Large doses of vitamin C can cause diarrhea if you're unaccustomed to them.

Fish oil for essential fats

Fish oil is one of the only concentrated forms of essential fats. Essential omega-3 fats are powerful, natural, anti-inflammatory agents, and they help repair nerve and brain cells, regulate the immune system, and even improve mood.

Typical dosage is 1 to 3 grams of distilled fish oil daily. Buy fish oil capsules that have been molecularly distilled to remove toxins like mercury, pesticides, and PCBs. You can find a current list of recommended brands at www. BeatingSugarAddiction.com.

If you experience stomach upset or fishy burps, try an enteric-coated capsule. If you're allergic to fish, you can use krill oil instead.

Fish oil has a mild blood-thinning effect. If you use prescription blood thinners like Warfarin or Plavix, consult a knowledgeable pharmaceutical professional before supplementing with fish oil.

Whey protein to help stabilize blood sugar

Powdered whey protein is the most efficient protein source available. Eating protein slows down the insulin response when you eat (which is good) and helps maintain blood sugar levels after you eat. Eating enough protein is one of the primary ways to keep the carb cravings away!

Whey protein contains *immunoglobulins,* which boost the performance of your immune system. Whey protein also has a high concentration of *glutamine,* an amino acid that's a vital component of the immune system.

Folks often report to me that one of their challenges is getting a protein source every time they eat. Whey protein is a quick and easy way to get your protein — add a scoop to your oatmeal, put it in your smoothie, or whip up a protein shake for a snack.

Choose a *whey protein concentrate* supplement that has no added carbohydrates, artificial colors, or artificial sweeteners. You can find a list of recommended brands at www.BeatingSugarAddiction.com.

Probiotics: The good bacteria

Humans have lots of different types of bacteria (sometimes referred to as *intestinal flora*) in the digestive tract, and these bacteria are an integral part of both the digestive and immune systems. The intestinal flora also keeps other insidious things from colonizing in the gut.

These beneficial bacteria are often killed off from antibiotics, poor diet, or stress. This is a major problem because a lack of beneficial bacteria in the gut can cause a host of problems with both digestion and immunity.

Taking a probiotic supplement is an easy way to help maintain the proper levels of favorable bacteria in your body. These are small capsules containing billions of helpful organisms to improve lactose intolerance, regulate bowel movements, improve symptoms of inflammatory gastrointestinal conditions (IBS, colitis, Crohn's), erase eczema, improve your immune system response, and clear up ulcers from *Helicobacter pylori* bacteria.

Typical probiotic capsules contain between 1 and 3 billion active organisms. For general health and immune system support, a daily dose of 1 to 5 billion organisms is generally sufficient. If you're combating a yeast infection, replenishing the gut after a course of antibiotics, or using probiotics for another therapeutic function, you may have to temporarily use a larger dose of 10 to 30 billion organisms per day. Consult a knowledgeable healthcare provider for advice.

Some probiotic supplements contain only two or three strains of bacteria. A more effective choice is a brand that contains many different strains.

Green drinks for extra vegetables

One of the difficulties reported to me on a regular basis is getting enough vegetables in the diet. A powdered green drink is a great way to put some more *phytonutrients* (plant nutrients) into your daily diet. I start every day with a glass of MetaGreens or Super Green Food.

Dozens of companies sell vegetable and fruit powder. Be sure to choose one without added sugars, fillers, or artificial sweeteners. A good green drink should include lots of different plants, such as alfalfa, aloe, barley grass, broccoli, dandelion leaf, ginger root, kale, nettle leaf, nopal cactus, oat grass, parsley, shave grass (horsetail), spinach, and wheat grass.

If you like to juice vegetables yourself, be sure to vary your concoctions from day to day so that you get a wide variety of nutrients in your diet (more about that in Chapter 6).

Magnesium for relaxed muscles and strong bones

Low levels of magnesium can make muscles shorten and spasm, causing achiness or muscle cramps. Magnesium relaxes muscles, improves sleep, and relieves tension.

According to a study published in *Diabetes Care,* magnesium deficiency can contribute to obesity and insulin resistance. High magnesium intake gives you a 30 percent less chance of developing metabolic syndrome too.

Magnesium helps keep your blood pressure normal and your heart rhythm steady. It's also a crucial mineral in the formation of bone tissue — anyone using a calcium supplement for osteoporosis should be sure that the supplement also contains magnesium (along with vitamin D, boron, and vitamin K2).

Studies show that overweight adults over age 40 who consumed less than 50 percent of the recommended amount of magnesium were twice as likely to have increased systemic inflammation, which contributes to major health problems such as heart disease, diabetes, and cancer.

Magnesium is also involved in the production of the three "happiness" neurotransmitters: serotonin, dopamine, and norepinephrine.

The recommended dosage of supplemental magnesium is 200 to 400 milligrams per day. Look for magnesium gluconate, magnesium aspartate (or another amino acid chelate), or magnesium citrate.

Chapter 6

Stocking a Low-Sugar Kitchen

. . . .

In This Chapter

▶ Creating a sugar-free kitchen

▶ Keeping good sources of protein and the right carbs on hand

▶ Making a grocery list and reading nutrition labels

▶ Eating healthier foods on a budget

. . . .

*A*s much as I hate to resort to clichés, when it comes to an eating plan, if you fail to plan, you plan to fail. Your kitchen is the control center of your nutrition universe; it's where you plan, store, and create the foods that make or break your eating system. If you don't stock your refrigerator and pantry with nutritious food from which to feed yourself and your family, you leave yourself and your loved ones at the mercy of chemical-laden convenience foods and perilous takeout packages. Planning and purposeful eating are the cornerstones of beating sugar addiction, and your kitchen needs to be an organized nutrition sanctuary for you to maintain long-term success.

This chapter is full of information to help you perform a total kitchen makeover. You find suggestions for how to stay organized and prepared and for what kinds of healthy foods you should stock in your refrigerator, pantry, and freezer. I tell you what to buy at the store and show you how to decipher the nutrition facts labels. You also discover how to identify some of the hidden sources of sugars in many common foods, and you find out when spending a little extra on organic and local food is worth the money.

Cleaning Out the Cabinets, Fridge, and Freezer

Everyone is a creature of habit, and the overloaded schedule that most people struggle with demands convenient and time-efficient meals. To successfully implement an improved eating plan, you must make sure that healthy, low-sugar foods are available in your house. If your kitchen and pantry are filled with junk food, your overloaded brain will drive you there when you finally take a moment to eat something. You're most likely going to eat whatever is handy, so the first step in upgrading to a healthier kitchen is to remove the junk food and stock a supply of quality food instead. Your goal is to make eating healthy food easy for you to do on a consistent basis.

Tossing the obvious culprits

If you don't keep junk food in your house, you won't have to worry about resisting the temptation to dive in! Get rid of these obvious sugar culprits:

- Agave nectar
- Baked treats like cakes, pies, Danishes, donuts, and pastries
- Candy
- Cookies
- Honey
- Sodas and other sweetened drinks, including juice drinks, diet sodas, prepackaged tea drinks, and energy drinks
- Syrup
- Table sugar

Next, look at the labels on the jars in the pantry and fridge. Toss (actually, empty and recycle) bottles or sauces whose first or second ingredient is "sugar" or ends with "syrup" — corn syrup, rice syrup, or agave syrup, for example.

If you'd like to take things a step further or if you're dealing with blood sugar problems like diabetes, you can also remove white flour products (look at the ingredients and toss anything whose first ingredient is "enriched").

Uncovering less-obvious troublemakers

Sugar is prevalent in the Western food supply, and it comes in many forms, with many different names. Cutting back on how much sugar you eat isn't always easy if you're not aware of how sugars can be disguised on the list of ingredients. When you're looking at labels and deciding what to keep or discard, consult the nearby sidebar "Other names for sugar" and Chapter 3 for many alternative names for sugar.

The first place to look when seeking out hidden sugar is in foods that are otherwise considered healthy. Though fruit juice, protein bars, and granola have more nutrients than empty-calorie junk food, if you look at the nutrition facts you'll find that most of them are laden with sugars. The fact that a food contains vitamins and antioxidants doesn't make it sugar-free!

Fruit juice and juice drinks

Fruit juice contains a lot of concentrated fructose because none of the fruit pulp or fiber is present. Concentrated fructose is a direct path to obesity and diabetes, so while 100 percent fruit juice may be high in vitamins and antioxidants, you should drink it sparingly, if at all. If you do drink fruit juice, limit your serving to 4 ounces at a time (that's half a glass).

Juice drinks, juice cocktails, and juice boxes marketed for children are required to contain only 10 percent actual fruit juice. The rest can be (and usually is) high-fructose corn syrup or another manufactured sweetener. Juice drinks are far worse than real fruit juice because they have all the calories and fructose but none of the nutrients of natural fruit juice. Juice boxes may also be loaded with artificial coloring and preservatives.

Diet drinks

Even though a diet soda shows zero calories and zero sugar on the label, you should stay away from these poisonous beverages. Chemical sweeteners are proven health hazards and appetite stimulants (see Chapter 3), artificial caramel coloring is a carcinogen, and the phosphoric acid in soda leaches calcium out of your bones. Soda, whether sweetened or unsweetened, doesn't have a single redeeming quality, so stay away!

If you love the fizz of soda, drink mineral water flavored with a slice of lemon or lime instead.

As you work to wean yourself off sugar, consider using *stevia powder* as a low-calorie sweetener instead of NutraSweet, saccharin, or any other chemical concoction. Be sure to read the label to confirm that the brand of stevia you buy has no added sugars or artificial sweeteners.

Other names for sugar

When you're looking at labels and deciding what to keep or discard, be on the lookout for these common names for sugar:

- ✔ Barley malt
- ✔ Dehydrated cane juice
- ✔ Dextrose
- ✔ Evaporated cane juice

- ✔ Fructose
- ✔ Fruit juice concentrate
- ✔ Maltodextrin
- ✔ Molasses
- ✔ Sucrose

You can find a more complete list of alternative names for sugar in Chapter 3.

Skipping low-fat options

The United States went through a huge fat-free food craze in the 1990s. Because fat-free food was in demand, food manufacturers added sugar and other flavorings to make up for the taste of the missing fat. At the time, most people didn't think about calories or sugar content; they were only focused on cutting back on the number of fat grams they ate. As a result, the amount of sugar consumed annually by the average American has gone up by 40 pounds since 1990 (that's almost 21 pounds of extra body fat from sugar calories), and obesity rates have more than doubled since then!

Dietary fat is important for a host of vital functions in your body (see Chapter 5), including producing hormones, conducting nerve impulses, regulating your immune system, absorbing certain vitamins, and building cell membranes. Dietary fat has the important job of slowing down the breakdown of carbohydrates in your digestive system, so you get a smaller insulin response when you eat fat with your food. Low-fat, high-carb eating increases the amount of insulin that your body produces, leading to obesity and insulin resistance.

Fat has more calories per gram than carbohydrates or protein, so eating fat helps you feel full. As discussed in Chapter 3, eating a low-fat, high-carb diet puts you on the blood sugar roller coaster, stimulating your appetite and activating sugar cravings.

Not all fats are good fats. Stick with healthy monounsaturated fats from fish, oils, nuts, and seeds while minimizing inflammatory trans fats from hydrogenated oils and saturated fats from feedlot meat and dairy.

Eliminating questionable foods

When in doubt, throw it out (or donate it). All you really need to eat to be healthy is hormone-free protein; a large variety of organic vegetables and fruits; and some essential dietary fat (fish oil, nuts, olive oil, canola oil). Most of your food every day should be composed of these simple, natural items. If you're pulling your hair out trying to decipher labels and count sugar grams, stop fretting about the details and make things really simple for yourself: If it's not a protein, a plant, or a healthy fat, don't eat it, and don't buy it for your family. You have plenty of opportunities to consume sugar and chemicals when you're out and about, so don't keep that stuff in your house. If your day-to-day food is healthy and sugar-free, you won't have to split hairs when you're eating out at special occasions.

 If you're going to get rid of a lot of extra food that you don't want in the house any more, don't waste it. You can find a local food bank at `http://` `feedingamerica.org` or donate to a local soup kitchen found at `www.` `foodpantries.org`.

Creating a Sugar-Smart Kitchen

The keys to staying on track with a healthy eating system are to plan ahead and to make sure that healthy foods are available and convenient. After you use the guidelines in the preceding section to remove the sugar-infused garbage from your pantry, refrigerator, and freezer, it's time to refill them with upgraded food choices.

Stocking up on protein

Protein and vegetables are your two best friends when it comes to staying sugar-free. Protein slows down the absorption of carbohydrates into the bloodstream and helps you feel satisfied for longer periods of time. Protein is important for a myriad of other functions in your body, which you can read about in Chapter 5.

A sugar-smart kitchen should have two main sources of protein handy:

- Wild-caught fish and pasture-raised meat and eggs in the freezer and refrigerator for planned meals.

- Powdered whey protein for last-minute snacks or for whenever you need a handy source of additional protein. Visit `www.BeatingSugar` `Addiction.com` for current brand recommendations.

Tips for buying and cooking healthy fish

Whenever possible, you should buy fish that's wild-caught instead of farmed. According to data from the U.S. Department of Agriculture, farmed fish are clearly inferior to their wild counterparts from both a nutritional and environmental perspective:

✔ Farm-raised fish contain much higher amounts of pro-inflammatory omega-6 fats than wild fish.

✔ Farmed fish are typically raised in crowded commercial tanks and pens and are therefore prone to disease and parasites. Fish farmers add antibiotics and pesticides to their food, and even vaccinate them!

✔ Farmed fish contain less beneficial omega-3 fats than wild fish but have a much higher fat content by weight.

✔ Farmed fish meat contains far higher concentrations of dangerous chemicals like polychlorinated biphenyls (PCBs) and dioxins.

✔ Farmed salmon are fed a pink-colored dye to change the color of their flesh.

✔ Fish farming can have drastic effects on wild fish — 95 percent of wild fish will die if they contact water infested with a fish farm's sea lice.

✔ Wild salmon have an average of 20 percent more protein than farmed salmon — they're not artificially fattened like farmed salmon.

You can drastically reduce some of the contaminants in fish by cutting off the skin and fat before cooking. Broil or grill fish on a rack so the fat drips off the fish, and don't use fish drippings for sauces. Don't eat fish organs or the dark patches of fish meat, because more contaminants collect there.

To reduce the consumption of mercury in fish, avoid eating large predatory fish like shark, swordfish, or king mackerel. White tuna (larger fish) generally has more mercury than light tuna, although levels vary widely.

For more information about environmentally responsible seafood do's and don'ts, visit `www.montereybayaquarium. org/cr/cr_seafoodwatch/sfw_ recommendations.aspx`.

When you make your food plan for the next day or two (or for the week), be sure to make notes about when to move frozen meats into the refrigerator so they're thawed when it's time to cook them.

I recommend buying meats from local farmers so you can talk to them firsthand about how they raise their livestock. It's also important to support local agriculture and community farms. See the "Eating local: Farmers' markets" section later in this chapter for more info.

Finding the right carbs

Most of the carbohydrates you eat should come from vegetables. Vegetables are low in calories and sugar and high in nutrients and fiber. You can pretty much eat all the veggies you want without having to worry about calories or insulin response.

To make vegetables easily available in your kitchen, keep your refrigerator stocked with fresh, crunchy produce ready to steam or eat raw. When fresh vegetables aren't in season from local farms, you can buy frozen vegetables for quick and easy cooking or pick up a bag of prewashed organic salad mix.

I don't recommend that you use canned vegetables because they're often high in sodium and can contain contaminants like bisphenol-a (BPA). In April 2012, the U.S. Food and Drug Administration (FDA) opted not to ban BPA from food and beverage containers.

To make vegetables easily available, keep a see-through container of raw, cut vegetables in the refrigerator. For a snack or an appetizer, dip raw, crunchy vegetables in olive oil or organic sour cream.

Here are some more tips for working more vegetables into your meal planning:

- ✔ Add steamed chopped vegetables to pasta or rice.
- ✔ Include a salad of mixed greens with your meal at least once per day.
- ✔ Plan some meals around a vegetable main dish, such as vegetable soup or a vegetable stir-fry.
- ✔ Shred carrots or zucchini into meatloaf, casseroles, and muffins.

Discovering satisfying beverages

One of the difficulties reported by many sugar addicts is staying away from soda (see the "Diet drinks" section earlier in the chapter). To transition away from sweetened drinks, you can start incorporating mineral water flavored with fresh citrus or investigate the endless varieties of teas you can brew.

Avoid drinking energy drinks, bottled teas, or sports drinks because they're usually loaded with sugar (or artificial sweeteners), caffeine, and chemical additives.

An easy way to reduce the frequency of sugar cravings is to make sure that you stay hydrated throughout the day. Make it your goal to drink at least 64 ounces of distilled water or mineral water each day. Use a stainless steel water bottle so you can easily measure and monitor how much water you drink.

Navigating the Grocery Store (And More)

You find most of the natural food that you should load up on — meats, fish, eggs, vegetables, fruits, and dairy products — along the outer perimeter of the grocery store. Processed and packaged foods generally make up a majority of the shelves in between. With the exception of nuts, legumes, and oils from the aisles, most of the selections in your shopping cart should consist of whole foods from the store's outer ring.

Making your list and sticking to it

Planning your meals in advance is a vital part of eating well and avoiding reactive eating. An integral part of executing your plan is maintaining your grocery list. Without the right supplies, you'll have a hard time providing quality nutrition for yourself and the rest of your family.

On your grocery list, keep a running list of all the items you need for the upcoming meals that you've planned. List some healthy snacks to have on hand, too. Don't forget to include healthy beverages like distilled water, mineral water, and green tea. Double-check the pantry for any ingredients you need for recipes, and be sure that you have enough staples like olive oil and butter on hand for cooking.

 When planning menus and making your grocery list, try to include vegetables in a variety of colors. Different colors indicate different phytonutrients, so make an effort to include red, green, orange, purple, and white plants (see Table 6-1).

Table 6-1	Fruit and Vegetable Color Chart
Target Color	*Example Foods*
Red vegetables and fruits	Tomatoes, red peppers, strawberries, cherries, cranberries, radishes
Green vegetables and fruits	Spinach, lettuce, green beans, broccoli, soybeans, green bell peppers
Orange/yellow vegetables and fruits	Banana peppers, oranges and tangerines, pineapple, lemons, carrots, papaya, yellow squash, winter squash
Purple/blue vegetables and fruits	Beets, blueberries, eggplant, currants, plums, purple onion, grapes, purple cabbage
White vegetables and fruits	Cauliflower, pears, garlic, mushrooms, onions

Table 6-2 shows some simple substitutions you can make on your grocery list to improve the quality of your food.

Table 6-2	Simple Grocery List Substitutions
Instead of This	*Buy This*
Commercial ground beef	Grass-fed ground beef or bison
Soft drinks	Mineral water
Sweetened bottled tea	Green tea bags
Seasoning packets	Fresh herbs, garlic, or onion powder
White rice	Brown rice or quinoa
Jif, Skippy, Peter Pan, or other peanut butter with sugar and hydrogenated oil	Natural peanut butter or almond butter
White bread	Spelt bread
White pasta	Brown rice pasta, corn pasta, or quinoa pasta

Reading and understanding food labels

The nutrition facts label is your key to uncovering the truth about the food inside. The nutrition facts label shows you the serving size, the calorie count, the basic nutrition breakdown (protein, carbs, fat, sugar, sodium, and so on), and, most important, the ingredients. See Figure 6-1 for an example of a typical nutrition facts label.

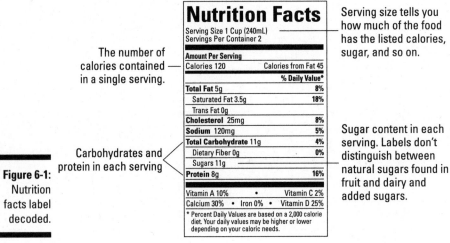

The number of calories contained in a single serving.

Serving size tells you how much of the food has the listed calories, sugar, and so on.

Carbohydrates and protein in each serving

Sugar content in each serving. Labels don't distinguish between natural sugars found in fruit and dairy and added sugars.

Figure 6-1: Nutrition facts label decoded.

Illustration by Wiley, Composition Services Graphics

Even though most of your healthiest meals consist of whole foods without labels, you should watch out for trouble on the nutrition labels of anything you buy that comes wrapped or boxed — bread, crackers, nuts, and condiments, for example.

Here are several things to watch out for on nutrition labels:

- **Enriched flour:** Even baked goods that prominently display *whole wheat* or *whole grain* on the packaging are often made of mostly enriched flour, with just a sprinkling of whole-grain flour added in. Read the ingredients list to see whether the primary flour is enriched flour, and look for products with organic whole-grain flours as the first ingredient instead.

- **High sugar content:** Replace any packaged food with more than 10 grams of sugar per serving with a lower-sugar alternative (the exception to this is unsweetened fruit, which contains more than 10 grams of natural sugar per serving). Note that the nutrition facts panel doesn't differentiate between naturally occurring sugars (such as those in fruit and dairy) and added sugars (such as high-fructose corn syrup). Be on the lookout for ingredients that appear in the "Other names for sugar" sidebar earlier in this chapter.

✔ **Trans fats:** If you see the word *hydrogenated* anywhere in the ingredients, put the item back on the shelf.

Pay attention to the serving size noted on the nutrition label of packaged foods. Measure out a serving to see how that compares to the amount that you normally eat; you may find that without checking, you ordinarily eat many servings' worth of calories and sugar!

Some food labels display claims or descriptions like *sugar-free* or *good source of fiber*. The FDA has specific requirements for food label claims, which are detailed in Table 6-3.

Table 6-3	Nutrition Content Claims
If the Label Says	*Then It Has This (per Serving)*
Low calorie	40 calories or less
Calorie free	Less than 5 calories
Low fat	3 grams or less of fat
Fat free	Less than ½ gram of fat
Low saturated fat	1 gram or less of saturated fat
Low cholesterol	20 mg or less of cholesterol and 2 grams or less of saturated fat
Cholesterol free	Less than 2 mg of cholesterol and 2 grams or less of saturated fat
Low sodium	140 mg or less of sodium
Very low sodium	35 mg or less of sodium
Sugar free	Less than ½ gram of sugar
Good source of fiber	2.5 grams or more of fiber
Lean (meat, poultry, and seafood)	Less than 10 grams of total fat, 4.5 grams of saturated fat, and 95 mg cholesterol
Extra lean (meat, poultry, and seafood)	Less than 5 grams of total fat, 2 grams of saturated fat, and 95 mg of cholesterol
High, rich in, or excellent source of	Contains 20% or more of the daily value
Good source, contains, or provides	Contains 10–19% of the daily value
More, fortified, enriched, added, extra, or plus	10% or more of the daily value; may only be used for vitamins, minerals, protein, dietary fiber, and potassium

3-in-1 healthy meal planning

My clients often state that the primary reason they don't eat better is that they don't have time to cook every day. If you struggle with finding time to cook, this 3-in-1 meal planning system may be just the trick! The basic idea is that you cook once and then use whatever you made for two (different) subsequent meals. For example, prepare grass-fed beef tenderloin for dinner one night, and then use the leftovers for sandwiches and soup on subsequent days. Here are some more examples using chicken and salmon:

3-in-1 Chicken

✔ Day 1: Roast a chicken (rosemary with vegetables is my personal favorite).

✔ Day 2: Use the leftover chicken to make a Mexican enchilada by wrapping it up with some sautéed onions, melted cheese, sour cream, and lettuce/tomato. This takes less than five minutes to make.

✔ Day 3: Pull the remaining chicken off the bones and sprinkle it in a mixed green salad.

3-in-1 Salmon

✔ Day 1: Bake a big piece of wild-caught salmon (you can use the Honey Dijon Salmon recipe in Chapter 15).

✔ Day 2: Make salmon cakes! (You can find a gazillion recipes on the Internet.)

✔ Day 3: Make salmon stir-fry by adding the remaining salmon to fresh veggies and wild rice in your favorite sugar-free sauce. Your vegetable chopping time is only a minute or two, and the cooking time is only six minutes.

Eating local: Farmers' markets

The grocery store isn't the only place where you can find healthy food. Farmers' markets offer great opportunities to get fresh, organic, locally grown foods. Actually meeting the farmers who deliver food into your community is an easy way to ascertain the origin of your food (and to verify the farming methods used to produce it) and to become more actively involved in your own nutrition. Doing so also provides a great opportunity to teach your children the importance of being proactive about healthy eating.

You can visit www.localharvest.org and http://search.ams.usda.gov/farmersmarkets to find farmers' markets, family farms, community-supported agriculture organizations (CSAs), and other sources of organic and sustainably grown food in your area.

Considering feedlot meat versus pasture-raised meat

Regardless of whether you decide to buy organic produce, if you eat meat I strongly recommend that you choose pasture-raised beef and chicken. Animals that are pasture-raised are much healthier because they have access to their natural diet and get plenty of exercise and sunshine. Animals raised in conventional feedlot operations are confined to overcrowded pens where, instead of their natural diet, they're fed genetically modified grains and given large doses of antibiotics and growth hormones.

As you may imagine, an animal's diet has an enormous impact on the nutritional content of the meat from that animal. Scientific studies show that regular consumption of feedlot meat causes inflammation and increases the risk of heart disease and cancer. Grass-fed meat, however, has been shown to have less fat, higher vitamin and mineral content, a healthier ratio of omega-3 to omega-6 fatty acids, and higher concentrations of conjugated linoleic acid (CLA), a cancer fighter. Meat isn't bad for you — *bad* meat is bad for you!

If your health and the health of the animals aren't enough to sway you against feedlot livestock, you can make a strong environmental case against confined animal feeding operations, too. Fossil fuel consumption for the production and transportation of commercial feed adds millions of tons of carbon dioxide into the atmosphere every year. Feedlots continuously add mind-boggling amounts of animal waste, hormones, and pharmaceutical runoff into the groundwater. Antibiotic resistance is rampant from drugs added to livestock feed.

Organic beef isn't the same as *grass-fed beef.* Organic meat comes from animals that are raised without antibiotics or growth hormones and are fed an organic vegetarian diet (which may or may not include corn and grains). Grass-fed beef is meat from cattle raised solely on grass, hay, and forage.

Going Sugar-Free on a Budget

In general, whole food is more expensive than packaged convenience foods, and organic food costs more than industrial food products. The popularity of clean organic food is bringing the price down over time, but at present, sugar and chemicals are unfortunately still cheaper than quality food. You can take some steps, however, to make sugar-free or low-sugar nutrition more affordable.

Stretching your grocery dollars

If you find yourself on a very tight food budget, here are some tips to get the most for your money without resorting to junk food:

✔ Check local newspapers, grocery websites, coupon sites, and in-store specials and coupons. Ask about a loyalty card for extra savings at stores where you shop. Meat and seafood are often the most expensive items on your list, so when you find a good deal, buy extra and stock the freezer.

✔ Other than items you can freeze, don't buy too much food at one time. Produce and fresh meat only keep for a few days in the refrigerator, so don't buy more than you can use in the next two or three days.

✔ Don't shop when you're hungry! Stick to your list, and try to be at the grocery store when you're not too rushed so you can make smart decisions.

✔ Check the "sell by" dates and be sure that you pick the freshest option. Grocery stores don't always rotate stock reliably.

✔ Instead of deciding on a meal and then buying the ingredients for it, try reversing the process and seeing what healthy meals you can invent using what you already have in the house.

✔ Stretch expensive meats into more portions by using them in meals like stews, casseroles, and stir-fry.

✔ Buy produce locally in season — it's not only less expensive but also fresher and a better environmental choice.

Knowing when to buy organic

My personal preference is to buy organic food whenever possible. In my opinion, not being exposed to pesticides, herbicides, chemical fertilizers, and genetically modified plants is totally worth the extra money. Plus, I think it's important for society as a whole to support farmers who use chemical-free, environmentally responsible methods.

Understandably, not everyone is willing or able to commit to organic food full time. Sometimes your food budget may require that you buy less-expensive conventional produce instead of organic foods. If that's the case, don't worry — the benefits of a diet that's high in vegetables and fruits outweigh the risks from pesticide use and genetically modified food. If you have to prioritize, go with organic when you buy foods that have been shown to accumulate high concentrations of pesticides — affectionately known as the *dirty dozen*.

Conversely, you can feel okay about buying the conventionally grown produce on the *clean 15* list because it's typically less contaminated. Table 6-4 presents both lists, which come from data from the U.S. Department of Agriculture.

Table 6-4	The Dirty Dozen and the Clean 15
Dirty Dozen: Buy Organic	*Clean 15: Conventionally Grown Is Okay*
Apples	Asparagus
Bell peppers	Avocado
Blueberries	Cabbage
Celery	Corn (non-GMO)
Cucumbers	Domestic cantaloupe
Grapes	Eggplant
Lettuce	Grapefruit
Nectarines	Kiwi
Peaches	Mango
Potatoes	Mushrooms
Spinach	Onions
Strawberries	Pineapple
	Sweet peas
	Sweet potatoes
	Watermelon

The lists in Table 6-4 assume that you rinse or peel fresh produce. Rinsing reduces but doesn't eliminate pesticides. You can use a vegetable wash to help remove even more chemicals. I don't recommend peeling because peeling removes valuable nutrients along with the skin.

Chapter 7

Sugar Detox 101

· ·

In This Chapter

▶ Understanding the myriad benefits of a sugar detox

▶ Getting started on your detox journey

▶ Checking out complementary medicine therapies and practitioners

· ·

*D*etox and *cleanse* are two terms that are often used to indicate a dietary plan that reduces or eliminates consumption of unhealthy substances. Whether you take a step-by-step approach to gradually reduce your sugar intake or you quit sugar cold turkey, you'll reap the benefits of detoxifying your body from the harmful effects of sugar overload.

This chapter helps you appreciate all the mental, physical, emotional, and medical benefits of getting off sugar — many of which you may never have thought of. I also give you a few tips on finding some holistic medicine options that may assist your quest to detox from sugar.

Appreciating What a Sugar Detox Can Do for You

Sugar, in excessive amounts, is one of the most harmful substances you can eat. When you look at a piece of candy, a soda, or a bag of pastries, you may not think of the word *toxin,* but refined sugars (along with other artificial sweeteners) place a huge physiological stress on your body's systems. Only smoking can match sugar's long-term damage to the body. High blood sugar levels cause damage to blood vessels and organs, and high insulin levels promote fat storage. Sugar makes your immune system less effective and creates a strong inflammatory response throughout the body. Getting off sugar can end all that!

Is going cold turkey best for you?

I generally advocate a gradual approach to sugar reduction because a drastic, overly strict eating regimen isn't a sustainable system for most people. However, I do occasionally encounter an individual for whom a rigid, cold-turkey approach to quitting sugar works best.

If you decide to stop eating sugar cold turkey, treat yourself like you're in detox for an addiction to narcotics. The first week of sugar abstinence is the hardest because that's when the cravings are the most powerful. Be gentle with yourself in other areas of your life — this isn't the time to tackle a large project, implement lots of other life changes, or work overtime. Give yourself extra support by going to bed early, taking naps when you need them, and cooking simple, nourishing meals. Spend quiet time in prayer or meditation. Call on others for support and encouragement when you need it (see Chapter 11 for advice on building a support system).

Detoxing from this inflammatory devil gives you a jump-start down the road toward weight loss, improved energy, better immune system function, and superior nutrition. A simple sugar detox can also quell your cravings for sweets, improve your mental clarity, and lead you toward a more empowered and fulfilled life.

The best way to rid your body of toxins is to avoid them in the first place. An ounce of prevention is worth a pound of detox! Read through Chapter 3 for an understanding of sugar and carbohydrates and how to find hidden sources of sugar.

Aiding weight loss

When you stop feeding yourself empty sugar calories, and when your insulin levels aren't elevated from eating too many carbohydrates, you begin to lose weight. More specifically (and more importantly), you begin to lose body fat.

Body fat is toxic. *Adipocytes* (fat cells) secrete inflammatory proteins that contribute to cardiovascular disease, arthritis, Alzheimer's disease, fibromyalgia, and other diseases brought on by chronic inflammation. Body fat cells are also storehouses for toxins in your body. Many substances that your kidneys and liver can't metabolize — pesticides, polychlorinated biphenyls (PCBs), and poisonous metals like lead and mercury — are tucked away and stored in fat cells (in the toxicology field, this is referred to as *bioaccumulation*).

Detoxing from sugar gives you a powerful head start toward shedding toxic body fat.

Achieving better blood sugar and insulin control

Excessive sugar or other carbohydrates elevates blood sugar levels and triggers an overproduction of insulin (consult Chapters 3 and 5 for more information on carbohydrates, insulin, and glycemic load). Chronically high insulin levels lead to obesity and diabetes. Detoxing from sugar stops the insulin roller coaster and helps level out your blood sugar levels, which is critical to avoiding (or reversing) diabetes.

Experiencing increased energy

When your blood sugar levels are stable, you don't experience the post-insulin sugar crashes that cause fatigue and brain fog. Less sugar in your diet helps keep your energy high, especially if you get some consistent exercise (see Chapter 12 for the lowdown on exercise).

In addition to smoothing out your blood sugar levels, detoxing from sugar helps coax your thyroid and adrenal glands back to their normal function, so you'll no longer suffer from the overwhelming fatigue that afflicts so many sugar addicts. You can read more about how sugar affects your hormones and endocrine system in Chapter 4.

Getting more nutrients

Sugar, along with many other sweeteners like high-fructose corn syrup, contains zero nutrients, only calories. When you eat sugar, you consume calories without nutrition, and this leads to weight gain, malnutrition (even if you're too fat), and cravings.

When you start replacing empty sugar calories with higher-quality carbohydrates like vegetables and fruits, you dramatically increase the amount of essential vitamins, minerals, and phytonutrients in your diet. Your body requires these vital nutrients to stay vibrant and to prevent all manner of diseases and illnesses. Better nutrition leads to a healthier body and fewer sugar cravings, too! See Chapter 5 for an overview of healthy nutrition basics.

Improving immunity

Dumping a large amount of sugar into your stomach lowers your immune system's effectiveness by about 30 percent for several hours. Consistent sugar consumption keeps your immune system permanently depressed. A sugar detox allows your immune system to leap back to full function.

Another important component of the immune system is the intestinal flora. The good bacteria in your gut stimulate the production of immune cells and play a major role in metabolizing dietary carcinogens. A high-sugar diet kills off the intestinal flora, compromising your immune system and allowing foreign pathogens (like yeast) to flourish. Detoxing from sugar and using a quality probiotic supplement (see Chapter 5 for the skinny on probiotics) restores the intestinal flora to a healthy state. Visit www. BeatingSugarAddiction.com for recommended brands of probiotics and other nutrition supplements.

Reducing inflammation and lowering your risk of disease

The inflammatory response is a necessary part of your physiology. Your body uses controlled inflammation to heal wounds, fight infections, and rebuild muscles. But too much inflammation can lead to premature aging and major problems like atherosclerosis, eczema, arthritis, yeast infections, chronic pain, autoimmune disorders, Alzheimer's disease, and cancer.

Sugar is an inflammatory food, so if you eat sugar frequently you're placing your body in a continuously inflamed state. If you don't yet suffer from inflammation problems, getting off sugar now can help prevent the onset of some terrible diseases in the future. If you're currently battling one or more inflammatory conditions, detoxing from sugar will lower the inflammation in your body and help end the discomfort of irritable bowel syndrome, Crohn's disease, fibromyalgia, arthritis, and other conditions caused by chronic inflammation.

Having less gas

Sugar creates an acidic environment that kills the beneficial bacteria in the gut. Your body's good bacteria (the *intestinal flora*) are important for digestion, immune system function, and serotonin production.

Eating too much sugar alters the intestinal flora, and the sugar ferments in the intestines, leading to bloating and gas. Cutting back on your sugar intake reduces gas and diminishes that uncomfortable, bloated feeling.

Battling fewer cravings

Consistent sugar overdose wreaks havoc on your brain chemistry (see Chapter 4). If you're a sugar addict, the more sugar you eat, the more you want. Breaking the craving cycle is a big step in changing your eating habits for the better. As you start to wean yourself off sugar (or if you quit it cold turkey), you'll find that within a very short period, you no longer desire the sweet stuff. And if you do have some, you'll find that the sickly sweet goodies you used to dream about don't even taste good anymore.

To start overcoming your sugar cravings right away, flip to Chapter 9 to investigate identifying triggers and to start using the flowchart for what to do when a craving strikes.

Enjoying better skin

The inflammation from a high-sugar diet makes your skin prone to unsightly pimples, eczema, and other breakouts. Sugar also damages collagen, causing your skin to become stiffer and less elastic. The more sugar you eat, the more tissue damage you cause and the more wrinkles you get. Staying away from sugar is one of the best things you can do for your skin.

Sharpening mental clarity

In addition to physically damaging your brain, a sugar binge can cause a host of brain performance problems. Sugar addicts commonly suffer from a sugar "hangover," with symptoms like brain fog, fatigue, headaches, or emotional swings.

Detoxing from sugar stops the sugar highs and crashes, keeping your energy more stable and your brain more functional throughout the day. You'll sleep better too!

Feeling personal empowerment

One of the most powerful and life-changing rewards of beating sugar addiction (or any addiction) is the thrill of empowering yourself and running your life proactively, so that you're in charge of your own behavior. To make a blanket generalization, addicts tend to use external substances to supply them with the brain chemistry they desire. When you detox from whatever substance you've been using as a substitute for a healthy emotional state — in this case, sugar — you'll live a happier and more peaceful life, and your body will thank you for healing it after sugar's harmful onslaughts.

When you overcome sugar addiction, you take a giant step forward toward creating or improving other positive things in your life — relationships, exercise, career issues, time management, and self-care. When you start taking control of your attitude and your actions instead of living reactively from the stresses of the world, there's no end to the wonderful things you can accomplish for yourself and for others!

Taking Your First Detox Steps

Sugar detox is simply the act of stopping the ingestion of harmful amounts of sugar so that your body can begin to heal itself by de-acidifying your blood and tissues, shedding excess body fat, and coaxing your hormone and energy systems back to normal, healthy function.

Follow these tips to ensure success when you begin detoxing from sugar:

- ✔ **Create a list of reasons you want to live differently.** Common reasons are to become healthier, to regain control of your life, to overcome diabetes, to have more energy, or to lose weight, but you may have other personal reasons why you want to quit sugar. Be sure to list the *whys* and not the *shoulds* — to stay on track, it's very important to have personal, meaningful reasons for wanting to change.

- ✔ **Cut your sugar portions in half.** Unless you really need to quit sugar cold turkey, start a gradual sugar reduction plan by cutting your typical sugar intake in half.

- ✔ **Drink at least 64 ounces (eight 8-ounce glasses) of water each day.** Water helps keep sugar cravings at bay (see Chapter 5).

- ✔ **Eliminate sugar from your pantry and refrigerator.** You can't eat what you don't have! Keeping your household free of junk food makes it difficult to impulsively grab sugary snacks. Consult Chapter 6 for tips on performing a healthy kitchen makeover.

- ✔ **Redefine dessert.** You don't have to swear off desserts forever to get off sugar! Usually a bite or two of fresh fruit or dark chocolate satisfies your desire for something sweet at the end of a meal. See Chapter 17 for low-sugar dessert ideas.

- ✔ **Start getting some regular exercise.** A good workout burns calories, increases your energy, boosts your mood, tones your muscles, and increases your bone density and insulin sensitivity. Flip to Chapter 12 for tips on setting up a basic exercise program.

- ✔ **Stay away from sweetened drinks.** Sweetened beverages are a huge source of empty calories (see Chapter 3), and diet drinks made with artificial sweeteners carry some significant health hazards. Make water, tea, or mineral water your drink of choice.

Big Pharma's influence on your doctor

Sometimes traditional physicians (known as MDs) unfairly get a bad rap because of the poor track record that Western medicine has concerning improving the health status of its patients (see the statistics on the rise of obesity, diabetes, and healthcare costs in Chapter 4). In my experience, most MDs are well-intentioned professionals who do their best to help their patients using the training they've received.

Many doctors aren't receptive to (or educated about) nonpharmaceutical treatments, but it's not their fault. Physicians today are totally engulfed by the influence of pharmaceutical companies. Drug companies fund most of the research published in the major medical journals and pay speakers at medical seminars. Drug companies woo physicians with dinners and even vacations! Doctors have an incessant line of pharmaceutical reps lined up to see them at their offices. Because physicians learning about treatments that don't involve prescription drugs isn't in the drug companies' interest, they bombard the poor doctors with pro-drug, anti-alternative information and agendas.

Using Complementary Medicine for More than Just Detoxing

Because a lifetime of sugar abuse can cause significant damage to the body, some sugar addicts struggle with serious medical conditions resulting from years of an abusive diet. Improving your diet and getting some regular exercise are great first steps toward improving your health, but you may consider widening the scope of your health improvements to include stress management, personal growth, and holistic medical care.

Conventional medicine — prescribing prescription drugs — hasn't proven to be very effective in improving the health and well-being of those who struggle with nutrition and lifestyle issues; these drugs don't have an impressive track record for assisting people with stress, anxiety, or emotional wellness. Drugs can come with harsh side effects, too. Because doctors generally prescribe these prescription medications to treat lifestyle diseases, you may get more comprehensive advice about improving your health through nutrition and lifestyle changes by building a team of complementary medicine providers around you. *Complementary medicine* (sometimes called *integrative medicine* or *holistic medicine*) is a catchall term used to describe a method of patient care that combines conventional Western medicine with complementary treatments such as nutrition supplements, acupuncture, massage therapy, yoga, and stress reduction techniques.

Don't get me wrong — I'm not downplaying the value of Western medicine. All legitimate medical practices — both traditional and holistic — have their place, but the traditional doctor/hospital/Big Pharma system doesn't do a very good job of actually making people healthy. You must take personal responsibility for educating yourself and for developing the lifestyle habits that will keep you (and your family) healthy. Discovering a more well-rounded system of medical care can get you started in the right direction and multiply the benefits of your sugar detox.

Exploring complementary medicine options

Complementary medicine strives to treat the whole person, not just the disease symptoms. Examples of some integrative medicine therapies that have proven to create positive patient outcomes are:

- ✔ Acupuncture
- ✔ Biofeedback
- ✔ Chiropractic
- ✔ Exercise programs
- ✔ Health coaching
- ✔ Massage therapy
- ✔ Meditation and mindfulness practice
- ✔ Mind-body therapies
- ✔ Naturopathic medicine
- ✔ Nutrition counseling
- ✔ Tai chi
- ✔ Yoga

Integrative medicine is no longer considered fringe because it has proven to be a smashing success in medical centers that have implemented it within their systems. The number of hospitals that now offer complementary therapies has more than tripled in the last ten years, and another one-fourth of hospitals say they plan to add complementary therapies in the future. Duke Integrative Medicine (www.dukeintegrativemedicine.org) and the Vanderbilt Center for Integrative Health (www.vcih.org) are pioneers in the field, serving as successful role models for other medical centers seeking to develop their own integrative medicine programs.

Finding a well-rounded doctor

If you're interested in making a concerted effort to maximize your physical and emotional wellness, detoxing from sugar is a good first step, but you can do much more. To make good overall health a top priority, you need to seek out doctors and other advisors who understand more than just the standard practices and ideologies of traditional medicine. Fortunately, you can find plenty of physicians and other healthcare providers who consider a wide range of treatments and health enhancements that aren't limited to prescription medications. *Naturopathic physicians* (NDs or NMDs) are doctors trained in the use of natural and alternative medical treatments. Though naturopathic physicians can and do utilize prescription drugs in their practices, their first choice for getting someone well is typically something other than a prescription pad. This, in my opinion, is a very good thing, because 80 percent of Western medical problems are lifestyle diseases — conditions like heart disease, elevated cholesterol, and diabetes that are the direct result of lifestyle choices and habits.

If you can't get a good recommendation for a qualified ND or an open-minded MD from your friends and colleagues, you can visit www.acam.org (the American College for Advancement in Medicine) or www.icimed.com (the International College of Integrative Medicine) for a list of local integrative medicine providers.

Avoiding snake oil

The alternative medicine and nutrition fields contain a whole lot of garbage. A quick Internet search for any medical condition yields a host of results for miracle cures, quackeries, and testimonials without a shred of research to back up those claims. You need to vet complementary and alternative medicine (CAM) practitioners and products very carefully because bogus practices and products can be not only a waste of time and money but also downright dangerous. Here are some tips to help you steer clear of shams and snake oil:

- ✔ **Avoid any therapy that promises that it's the only solution or cure to your problem.** Quality integrative medicine doesn't blindly advocate a single alternative approach while rejecting all conventional ones. If the practitioner or product you're investigating promises to be the be-all, end-all to your problem and automatically dismisses all conventional treatments, move on.

- ✔ **Ask your physician, physical therapist, chiropractor, nurse practitioner, or other health-minded individual whom you trust for a recommendation for the type of provider you seek.**

- ✔ **Call your local hospital and ask whether it keeps a list of reliable CAM practitioners in your area.**

- ✔ **Consult a qualified nutrition expert before choosing nutrition supplements.** Many worthless products are proffered to the masses every day, some nutrition supplements can have serious side effects or interactions, and the purity and labeling accuracy of nutrition supplements varies widely among manufacturers. You really need to consult with a knowledgeable professional to be sure that you have a safe and effective nutrition regimen in place.

✔ **Contact CAM professional organizations to get names of local practitioners who are certified and have proper training in their field.**

Letting go of some other ugly addictions

By purchasing this book, you've already demonstrated your interest in beating sugar addiction. The good news is that, after you develop the skills and the mind-set to defeat one addiction, you can apply the same skills and methods to rid yourself of other unhealthy habits, too!

If you find yourself saddled with any of the following unhealthy addictions, see whether you can find some similarities between the beliefs and mind-set you have about sugar and the ones you have about these other addictions. Some multi-addicts have found that their problem isn't actually the stuff to which they're addicted — it's their unhealthy thinking habits!

✔ **Caffeine:** If you're an Exhausted Addict (see Chapter 2), you may abuse caffeine as much as you abuse sugar. Stress and poor diet have beaten you down to the point where your adrenal function doesn't work without an external stimulant. To reverse this downward spiral, follow the advice in Chapter 5 concerning eating enough protein, drinking enough water, and supplementing correctly. You can start to wean yourself off caffeine by drinking half-caff coffee instead of full strength or you can begin drinking tea instead of more caffeinated beverages.

✔ **Smoking:** Though part of smoking addiction is chemical — nicotine creates a powerful physical addiction by stimulating feel-good chemicals like dopamine, serotonin, and adrenaline — another part of smoking addiction is *association*. Association is more of a behavior problem than a chemical addiction; people become attached to the "script" of having a cigarette when particular things happen, such as when a certain time of day arrives, when they consume certain foods or drinks, or when particular people are around them. If your smoking addiction has a strong *association* component, pick some positive substitute activities from Chapter 9 and find an alternative action to try whenever your "script" tells you it's time to light up. You may not be addicted to nicotine after all!

✔ **Victimhood:** The victim mind-set is often a strong driving force behind a person's substance abuse. Chronic victims usually exhibit woe-is-me attitudes, defensiveness, and strong inner critics masked by angry and judgmental behavior. Just like any addict, the victim gets mired in his or her story, but in this case ends up becoming addicted to being unhappy about being wronged.

If you're addicted to your victim mentality, changes in lifestyle and nutrition aren't enough to cure you — you need some professional help. Consult Chapter 11 for tips on finding support groups and qualified therapists, and visit www.BeatingSugarAddiction.com for recommended reading on changing your life by changing your thinking.

Part III
Living a Successful Sugar-Busting Lifestyle

Meal	Planned Time to Eat	Protein?	Vegetable?	Portion Check?	Insulin Check?
Oatmeal with whey protein	6:30 a.m.	✓		✓	✓
Greek yogurt with blueberries	10 a.m.	✓		✓	✓
Turkey wrap	1 p.m.	✓	✓	✓	✓
Celery boat with almond butter	4 p.m.	✓	✓	✓	✓
Grilled fish and steamed veggies	7 p.m.	✓	✓	✓	✓

Illustration by Wiley, Composition Services Graphics

web extras Discover the secrets of avoiding holiday weight gain at www.dummies.com/extras/beatingsugaraddiction.

In this part . . .

- ✔ Master mindful eating to control your portions and get more out of your eating experience, and kiss stress eating goodbye.

- ✔ Identify triggers that send you reaching for sugary foods.

- ✔ Know what to do when a craving strikes and sort out what your body really needs instead of sugar.

- ✔ Keep a level head when eating out at restaurants, parties, and special occasions.

- ✔ Surround yourself with a reliable support system and be prepared for how people may react to your change in lifestyle and eating habits.

- ✔ Increase your chance of success by including an exercise plan with the right balance of cardio and strength training.

Chapter 8

Eating Mindfully

*I*n counseling thousands of clients over the last 20 years, I've found that one theme reigns supreme: People have a hard time living purposefully instead of reactively because they feel that their lives are totally out of control. This mind-set can lead to a host of stress and anxiety disorders like sleep problems, weight gain, headaches, thyroid disease, panic attacks, auto-immune disorders, heart attacks, and cancer.

Chinese medicine has a word for this frantic, out-of-control mind-set — *xinyuan*, which translates, wonderfully, into "monkey mind." The term was adopted into Buddhist and Confucian teachings more than 1,500 years ago, but it has also become a popular term in modern psychology.

An uncontrolled monkey mind is the antithesis of a peaceful, happy, and fulfilled life. It's a serious detriment to your health and well-being, and it will wreak havoc on any dietary planning you attempt. To regain control of your life, you must learn to master your monkey mind.

Mindfulness is the key to quieting the monkey mind. This chapter lays out an explanation of mindfulness and how it relates to controlling your eating. I deliver tips on eating with intention, planning, and avoiding being obsessive about food. My goal in this chapter is to give you a crash course in living pro-actively instead of reactively so you can use those tools to create a healthy, sustainable eating plan to help you stay lean and craving-free forever!

What Is Mindful Eating?

Mindfulness is the act of being mentally and emotionally present, without judgment, while being aware of and intentional about your state of mind and your behavior. Basically, it means paying attention to what's happening without judging or reacting, and acting purposefully and intentionally.

Mindful eating requires that you pay attention to the cues your body gives you. It's easy to become fooled or distracted by external events, unhealthy habits, and unskillful reactions to the hiccups along the road of life. Eating mindfully means that you make food decisions based on the reality of what's happening right now, not on stories that you've told yourself for years or on the fantasy that shoveling sugar into your mouth will make your problems go away.

As you learn to pay attention to cues from your body, and as you practice making food decisions intentionally instead of reactively, you'll regain control over your eating style, and the careful attention and purposeful decisions will carry over to other aspects of your life. Mindful behavior of any type is a gateway to a more peaceful and empowered life!

Mastering Proactive versus Reactive Eating

It's very easy to turn to food, especially sugar, when you feel stressed or out of control. Sugar is pervasive in most of the world, and this cheap, readily available drug can exert harmful control over your life if you let it.

Proactive eating means that you don't allow these external cues to affect your eating behavior (what you choose to eat, when you eat, and how much you eat). Proactive eating decisions come from knowledge, planning, and consistent practice. Eating proactively is a skill that you must master to achieve lasting weight loss and to kick the sugar habit for good.

Here's a scenario that typifies unhealthy, reactive eating: After a long, stressful day at work, you come home late, too tired to cook something healthy for dinner. You plop down in front of the TV and begin munching on a bag of whatever you can grab out of the pantry. While you eat and watch, you also go through the mail, worry about this month's bills, and try to decide what you're going to wear to an event this weekend that you don't really want to go to anyway. When the bag is empty or when you feel disgusted with yourself for what you just ate, you finally stop eating . . . until you remember that you have ice cream in the freezer.

Examine some of the unmindful points of this scenario:

✔ You didn't plan ahead; dinner was an afterthought, and you ate whatever was handy. The pantry and freezer were stocked with unhealthy convenience calories.

✔ You paid no attention to the amount of food you ate. You can't control portions when you eat directly from a bag.

✔ You paid no attention to your body's cues. When you eat from a bag while doing several other things, you have very little awareness of any physical sensations or emotions. You have no idea when you've had enough to eat or why you're doing what you're doing.

✔ You didn't focus on any one task. The monkey mind stayed in full force the entire evening.

Here are some easy ways to improve the mindfulness of this situation:

✔ Eat enough during the day so that you're not starving when you get home.

✔ Keep your kitchen stocked with healthy food instead of convenience calories (see Chapter 6).

✔ Plan the day's food so that you don't have to think about what you're going to eat for each meal.

✔ Put your food on a plate before you start eating and take an honest look at what's there. Do you have vegetables? Where's your protein? What are the portions like? What's this meal going to do to your insulin levels? What can you do to improve the nutrition of this gift to yourself?

✔ While you're eating, savor the tastes and textures. Chew thoroughly. Pay attention to how your body feels so you know when you've had enough. The Japanese use the term *hara hachi bu,* which means "stomach 80 percent" — in other words, stop eating when you're 80 percent full.

✔ Stay focused on one task at a time. While you're eating, pay attention to that and only that. While you're watching a movie, focus. Pay full attention to the mail during commercials. When planning for future things, do so one at a time, using facts and strategy instead of reacting to anxiety and worry.

Paying Attention While You Eat

The practice of mindfulness is concerned with noticing (without judging) what's happening *right now.* That doesn't mean you can't think about the past or the future, but when you do, you should strive to do so without fear or judgment, and you shouldn't allow recognition of past events or future fears to dictate your behavior in the present.

Staying mindful is a skill that requires attention and practice. Without focus and attention on the present moment, the mind wanders to thoughts of the past or to worries about the future. This triggers all sorts of negative emotions like fear, anger, guilt, depression, and self-pity. If you indulge these kinds of thoughts, you reinforce their power in your life and the habits that you've built around them — most likely sugar abuse, if you're reading this book.

Eating with intention

Eating purposefully (instead of reactively) is the most important skill for controlling your weight and staying away from sugar. The lifestyle of modern society has created a host of external food cues that can easily override your body's natural cues about eating. While eating, instead of deciding whether they're still hungry, people typically use external cues to tell them when to stop. For example, an empty dinner plate is an external cue that it's time to stop. For most people, if a few bites of muffin remain in the wrapper or if a few soggy French fries are left at the bottom of the bag, they unconsciously decide that they must continue eating. People habitually eat as though their mission is to finish every last bite in front of them, because they were often forced to do this as children.

To stay mindful while you're eating, evaluate how you feel after every bite. Are you 80 percent full yet? Are you experiencing what you're eating or just chewing and swallowing mindlessly? Are you eating because you need nourishment or are you eating as a reaction to some external cue or habit?

Here are some tips to help avoid mindless eating situations:

- ✔ **Don't eat out of packages.** Put your portion on a plate or in a bowl and put the package away. If it's in front of you, you'll most likely eat it until it's gone.

- ✔ **Don't put serving dishes on the dinner table.** If you want more food, make yourself get up and go into the kitchen to get it.

- ✔ **Keep food out of sight.** Food that's visible (sitting out or in a glass container) gets eaten more, because every time you pass the candy jar at the office, you have to make a decision about whether to eat some. Every time you see it, you have to say "No" to something tasty and tempting. Eventually, the No's turn into, "Well, okay, just this once. . . ." Use "out of sight, out of mind" to your advantage.

> ✔ **Watch out for unconscious habits and scripts that dictate your behavior.** Beware of tricks like eating until the TV show is over or eating restaurant bread until the meal arrives.

> ✔ **You don't have to eat everything that's on your plate.** When you have more than protein and vegetables on your plate, don't feel obligated to eat it all. The first two bites of anything are the most satisfying.

Planning your food choices in advance

Many people fall victim to reactive eating because they're unprepared. If you don't know in advance what your food will consist of for the day, you're at the mercy of the cravings of your starving brain, which will drive you to grab whatever you can get quickly — and lots of it!

Eating on the fly with no plan is akin to investing in a company that has no budgets, where everybody says, "We just spend whatever we feel like from day to day and hope it all works out in the long run. Then we complain about how broke we are."

Plan your eating in advance, out to whatever time horizon suits you. I plan my next day's food the night before, but some folks prefer to lay out a week at a time so they only have to think about it once a week. Any time frame that works for you is fine, as long as you don't leave the house without knowing what you're going to eat for every meal and snack for the rest of that day.

Planning should include not only *what to eat* but also *when to eat* and *how much to eat.* Plan your eating times in your schedule as much as possible — doing so keeps you from going too long without food and succumbing to cravings and ravenous reactive eating.

Planning portions is easy if you prepare your own meals and snacks, but it can be tricky if you eat out a lot. At restaurants, avoid using the empty plate as the only measure of whether you're done eating. Look at the plate when it arrives and assess your portions using the list from Chapter 5. Consider putting half of your meal in a takeout container before you even start eating — chances are you'll be satisfied with half the amount. Eat vegetables first, then protein. After that, assess your 80 percent — do you need the extra starch or any more calories? Probably not.

Use the handy chart in Figure 8-1 to double-check your plan for the upcoming day. After listing the meal or snack and the time you plan to eat it, the chart has four columns for you to check off:

✔ Do you have a protein in the mix? See Chapter 5 if you need help with protein sources.

✔ Do you have vegetables at this meal? If you're bringing a sandwich for lunch, make sure it's loaded up with fresh lettuce, tomato, onion, peppers, or whatever other veggies you like.

✔ Have you considered your portions? Remember, no eating from packages or serving dishes. If you're planning on eating this meal out, be aware of your portions before you take the first bite.

✔ What will this meal do to your insulin levels? See Chapter 3 for information about your carbohydrate choices' effect on your insulin response. This is especially important if you have diabetes.

Meal	Planned time to eat	Protein?	Vegetable?	Portion check?	Insulin check?

Figure 8-1: Use this chart to plan ahead for meals.

Keeping a food journal (also known as a lie detector)

A food journal is one of the best tools for staying mindful and honest about how you're actually eating. After you eat something, write it down right away; at the end of a busy day, trying to remember what you had at what time (and how much of it) is asking for inaccuracy and denial. You should record every single thing that goes in your mouth besides water. If you bite it, you write it!

Research shows that dieters who keep a food journal lose more weight than those who try to improve their eating without one. In my experience, people tend to think they eat better than they actually do. When you record a few days of consumption, you may find that you're woefully short on vegetables or that you regularly eat way too many calories before bed. One bonus to keeping a food journal is that it makes you think more about what you choose and how much you eat. People generally report that keeping a food journal automatically improves their eating just by virtue of the fact that they have to think about it and write it down.

Visit www.BeatingSugarAddiction.com to download a basic food journal and to look over the recommended reading list for additional resources and guidance toward better mindfulness.

Avoiding being obsessive or neurotic about food

Being mindful and choosy about what you eat isn't the same as being obsessive or neurotic about food! Making smart choices from an informed and empowered position is desirable, whereas making decisions out of fear or deprivation can lead to guilt, resistance, overcompensation, and even eating disorders.

Food isn't your enemy, and you can't build a successful, healthy eating plan if you consistently act out of fear or resentment. To tell yourself that you'll never eat sugar again is unrealistic and shortsighted. Your goal should be to be better, not to be perfect. Any food plan that uses the word "never" is destined to lead to begrudging and bitter feelings, and ultimately, failure.

Obsessing over every tiny detail of your diet, being a control freak, and trying to be perfect are behaviors that stem from the fear of a lack of ability or personal power. Every time you find yourself at a decision point, remember that you're the decision-maker and the driver of your destiny. Empower yourself to make positive decisions in all phases of your life, and don't allow a fear of setbacks drive you to an obsessive or neurotic view of food.

Friends can provide an enormous amount of support on your quest to eat better (see Chapter 11), but obtaining assistance from a trained professional is often helpful. If you'd like to receive some professional help with mindful eating or if you have concerns about obsessive eating habits, consult the National Eating Disorders Association website at www.NationalEatingDisorders.org for information and treatment referrals.

Summoning willpower and understanding

Many people who struggle with sugar and weight control try to change their ways through deprivation diets, thinking that willpower is what they need. When their unsustainable plan goes awry, as it inevitably does, they tell themselves that they've blown it and give up completely.

From a mindfulness perspective, you never reach a point of no return; you can choose to eat mindfully at any time, even after blowing it for one meal or even for a whole month. People occasionally make choices they're not proud of. Own what you did (no excuses; it was your choice), recognize the effects that those behaviors have on your body, and make a plan to do something different next time.

Willpower is weak without an understanding of what you really want (see Chapter 9 for an important lesson about that). If you try to deny yourself the sugar that you're craving without stopping to think about why you're craving it, you'll eventually give in to the brain's cravings. And you'll have learned nothing and changed no behaviors or habits.

Willpower is sustainable when you use it as the discipline to get organized (and stay organized) and to act (and eat) purposefully and mindfully instead of reactively. If you bank on willpower to keep you away from sugar when you don't have planning and mindfulness in place, it will fail you.

Managing stress

One of the most reliable paths to sugar addiction and obesity is high stress, because stress changes your appetite, stimulates overeating, and increases insulin resistance.

Surveys show that a majority of women often eat for emotional reasons rather than hunger. Stressful emotions dampen the reward response in the brain, which causes cravings that drive overeating (and, for some people, the abuse of other substances, too). Stress affects the same signals as famine does: It turns on the brain's pathways that make people crave calorie-dense food (high fat and high sugar). The hunger and reward drives are some of the strongest in the human body, and they're very difficult to combat without the right tools.

Learning to turn the monkey mind into mindfulness is a lifelong practice, but here are a few simple stress management tips that can get you started:

- ✔ **Breathe.** Stopping to take a few deep belly breaths gives you a moment to gather your thoughts and become rational.

- ✔ **Empower yourself.** Remember that you're the one driving the bus. If you don't like where it's going, drive somewhere else! One of my favorite quotes by famous self-help author Wayne Dyer is, "Remember that you choose your attitude and your personality every second of every day."

- ✔ **Find meaning in what you do.** If your job is causing you stress, remember what you liked about your job when you started it. Consider what you may need to do differently to be satisfied in your position again.

Think about the necessity of your work, the purpose of your job, your personal goals, and the benefits that your work provides to others.

✔ **Identify the true source of your stress.** Stress comes from fear, so when you find yourself feeling overwhelmed or stressed out, take a moment to determine what you're afraid of. After you give yourself a reality check, you can determine whether your fears are well-founded. If they are, you can start taking appropriate action instead of just worrying.

✔ **Schedule something that you like to do that's just for yourself.** Take a walk, get a massage, read for fun, or take a nap. Be sure to put the activity on your schedule or you'll never get to it!

In Chapter 9, I help you identify triggers and choose substitute behaviors.

Giving yourself a reality check

It's easy to get overwhelmed by a busy life if you don't regularly pause for a reality check. Staying mindful helps you understand what's actually happening, what you're really afraid of, and what you really want.

When you find yourself faced with a negative emotion like anger, stress, or a sugar craving, ask yourself these three questions:

✔ What actually happened just before I reacted the way I did? Just the facts here — no blaming, assuming, or history allowed!

✔ What story am I making up (or what belief do I have) that led me to create the emotion I'm having?

✔ Because my story isn't true, what other attitude or emotion can I choose instead?

One of the greatest stress relievers is to uncover what a particular stressor or incident really means to you. For example, if you're feeling stressed out about work because you think you can't get everything done, ask yourself what not getting things done means to you. Does it mean that you're a failure? Do you think it means that you're unappreciated or misunderstood? Does it mean that you're unreliable or unlovable?

Find out what story you're telling yourself about what you think this thing that's freaking you out means to you. Shining the light of truth on your fears can uncover their blatant untruths or at least make them less scary.

If you haven't yet taken the quiz in Chapter 2, do so now and see whether one of the four typical behavior and psychology profiles fits your situation. Understanding the whys of your thoughts and behaviors helps keep your head on straight and gives you a powerful tool to stay on track with healthy eating habits.

An experiment in mindful eating

To get a feel for how mindful eating can enhance your eating experience, try this sequence the next time you're ready to sit down to eat something that you love. I use one of my personal favorites, cheese ravioli, for this example:

1. Before you do anything else, stop and be grateful for what you have and for what you're about to do.

2. Cut into a piece of the ravioli with a fork. Before you put anything in your mouth, notice what cutting perfectly cooked cheese ravioli feels like. Tune in to the texture of the pasta, observe and appreciate the cheese inside, and marvel at the bright color of the sauce in the bowl. Savor the aroma in the rising steam.

3. Place a forkful in your mouth. Feel the heat and the response that your mouth has.

4. Now comes the hard part — put the fork down. This is more challenging than you may think because that first bite feels and tastes so good, and the rest of the bowl is beckoning. You're hungry, after all! This experiment in eating, however, involves looking past the instinctive urge to plow into the rest of the bowl like a starving dog. Leave your fork on the table.

5. Chew slowly. No talking. Savor the texture of the pasta in your mouth and the contrast in flavors among the cheese, pasta, and sauce. How sweet, tart, or acidic is the sauce? Where do you feel it on your tongue? What are the sides of your mouth doing as you chew?

6. When you've chewed thoroughly and taken in all the new sensations you can for now, go ahead and swallow your first bite. What does it feel like as it passes through your throat? What happens in your stomach?

7. When you're done noticing, pick up your fork and cut another bite. Continue this way throughout the course of the meal and you'll experience the third eye–opening pleasures of the practice of mindful eating.

The concept of mindfulness has its roots in Buddhist teachings. Many Buddhist teachers encourage their students to meditate with food because it's an easy way to practice every day. Paying close attention to the sensation and purpose of each morsel expands your consciousness and appreciation. If you enjoyed this mindfulness experience with food, try practicing more mindful awareness during a walk after dinner!

Chapter 9

Breaking the Cycle of Failure and Staying On Track

● ●

In This Chapter

▶ Adopting new mind-sets and new habits

▶ Managing cravings

▶ Taking the right steps when you fall off the wagon

● ●

*N*o one should be expected to sustain an eating plan with zero fulfilling or enjoyable foods, and that includes you. This chapter talks about how to develop new habits and new ways of dealing with food without trying to remain on an unsustainable, restrictive "diet" (I hate that word!). I help you find your *new normal*, that all-important mind-set that guarantees you'll never again feel like you're on a diet.

Habits can be hard to change, and you won't always be perfect. If you're depressed or stressed, you may find yourself craving sugar or falling back into other unhealthy habits. This chapter helps you forgive yourself, deal with your inner critic, and get back in the driver's seat after a bad choice. Best of all, I show you exactly what to do when a craving strikes — a step-by-step system for staying on track!

Applying Strategies for Success

Everyone is different, but after 20 years of helping people overcome sugar addiction, I've identified some clear patterns. This section examines must-do strategies for success — vital skills to achieve the new habits and new mind-set you'll need to successfully break the cycle of sugar addiction.

As you pick up these principles and progress down the path of mindful eating, not only will you have more energy and feel much better, but your tastes will probably change. After a few weeks of nonaddictive eating, your desire for sugar is likely to drop dramatically!

Adopting a new mind-set

Any aspect of your life — your body, your relationships, your friendships, your attitudes — is strongly influenced by what you do most of the time. Whatever is "normal" for you yields a certain result. If you want to change some part of your life, you have to change what you usually do. You have to create a *new normal.*

The goal of any successful eating plan is to create a healthy, sustainable normal so that you're never on a diet or on a special plan; you just do things differently from how you used to do them. Improve your normal, and eating well will soon be just something that you usually do.

For many people, mindful eating seems to be one of the most challenging parts of revamping an eating plan, so you should expect to put some extra effort and attention into eating on purpose instead of reactively (Chapter 8 is all about eating mindfully).

When you find yourself craving something sweet (or when you have the urge for late-night snacking), check in with yourself to see whether food is what you're really after. Are you thirsty? Are you bored? Are you lonely or sad about something? You may find that you've established a habit of wanting something sweet anytime you feel *anything!* If you take a moment to acknowledge your true physical and emotional state when you think you want something, that habit isn't difficult to break.

Changing what's normal for you

Take a moment and write a sentence or two that describes what's currently normal for you in each of these circumstances:

✔ Breakfast

✔ Choice of snacks

✔ Eating frequency

✔ Food portions

✔ Late-night eating

✔ Planning your food (versus eating on the fly or eating whatever's handy)

✔ Vegetable intake

✔ Water intake versus other drinks

✔ What you do when you feel stressed

Take a close look at what you wrote. If you find that doing these things yields results that aren't working for you, use the tools in this chapter to start doing something different!

One more important thing to investigate for your new mind-set: You have to start looking at how you view food.

✔ Do you view food as your friend (maybe your only friend)? Your enemy?

✔ Do you use food as a reward? How about as a substitute for affection or mental stimulation? Have you been medicating yourself with sugar?

Here's your new mind-set: Food is nourishment. It's fuel for your body. You truly are what you eat. You need to start seeing food as that, and only that. Sure, eating has a social aspect, and the very act of eating can and should be an enjoyable and satisfying experience. But when you create stories in your subconscious mind about what food means to you, and when you use it as an unhealthy substitute for something else you need, it begins to hold a dangerous power.

Spend some time thinking about what stories you may be making up about sugar. For example, if you find yourself feeling overwhelmed and stressed, you may be telling yourself, "If I eat the rest of that ice cream, I will feel more peaceful and in control of my life." Huh? How can this possibly be true? When you come across a story you've been telling yourself about sugar, ask yourself, "Is this true?" I'll bet not — and hopefully you'll get a good laugh at the absurdity of the story, too!

Developing new habits

Sometimes the idea of changing your daily routines can seem daunting. When I interview new clients, they often report that in the past they felt overwhelmed by all the things they thought they had to keep track of when they tried to improve their eating habits. Don't despair! Developing new habits isn't as complicated or overwhelming as it may seem. Don't try to change everything at once, and don't think that from now on you have to eat perfectly all the time and deprive yourself of your favorite foods forever.

The following sections cover three simple habits you can adopt to stay on track with a quality eating plan.

Decide what and when to eat instead of eating reactively

The biggest challenge most people face is eating *purposefully* instead of *reactively*. To get off sugar and eat healthfully for the rest of your life, you need a new mantra: Decide, don't react! You must learn to eat with purpose. If you lose control over your food intake every time something unexpected or stressful happens in your life, you'll never be able to sustain a healthy eating system.

Plan ahead

Planning ahead is one of the most important habits you must develop to eat purposefully. Before you go to bed each night, take a minute and go through your meal planning for the next day. Write it down at first, especially if you find that you feel overwhelmed with planning meals in addition to everything else on your to-do list. Make sure that you're prepared for the day's eating schedule with this checklist:

- **Breakfast:** A breakfast high in protein helps control your blood sugar levels and staves off hunger more than a breakfast of all carbohydrates (cereal, waffles, bagels, toast, and so on). A protein-packed breakfast might include eggs from pasture-fed hens, hormone-free breakfast meats (sausage or ham), a whey protein shake, or some Greek yogurt. For more in-depth information on protein, see Chapter 5. You can find breakfast recipes in Chapter 13.

- **Snack:** To keep blood sugar levels stable and to avoid cravings, the best snacks combine a protein and a carbohydrate. Examples are an apple with almond butter, a cup of cottage cheese with some raw vegetables, or a homemade whey-and-vegetable-juice shake. See Chapter 3 for more information about blood sugar control and Chapter 16 for yummy, low-sugar snack recipes.

- **Lunch:** Don't forget to load up on the veggies at lunchtime! Here are a few good lunch examples:

  - A chicken or turkey sandwich or wrap with whole-grain bread and lots of green lettuce, tomatoes, spinach, olives, onions, peppers, or whatever other veggies you like. To minimize the amount of bread, try an open-faced sandwich with just one slice of bread.

  - A salad of mixed greens with grilled salmon and balsamic vinaigrette dressing.

  - Mixed vegetables and diced chicken sautéed in olive oil.

  You can find more low-sugar lunch ideas in Chapter 14.

- **Snack:** Like your morning snack, your afternoon snack should combine protein and carbohydrates. Many people find that something with desirable mouth feel helps keep them satisfied during the afternoon. If you like creamy, try Greek yogurt. If you like crunchy, try some apple slices or celery sticks with almond butter.

- **Dinner:** Be sure to have a healthy dinner planned, so you're not grabbing unhealthy convenience foods when you come home hungry after a long day. Having fresh fish or a turkey breast ready to cook allows you to put together a healthy, speedy meal. See Chapter 15 for some delicious dinner recipes.

✔ Be careful not to eat too much late at night, especially the starches. You should think about what you're going to do for the next four hours and plan your dinner accordingly. If all you plan to do after dinner is watch TV and go to bed, you don't need many calories! When you eat too much food before bed, you don't have a chance to burn off those calories, and they're simply stored as body fat.

In addition to the list of what you're going to eat, make sure you have

✔ Plenty of distilled water to drink throughout the day

✔ Any other approved sugar-free beverages you desire, like mineral water with citrus, or green tea

Obey the ten-minute rule

When a craving strikes, always wait ten minutes before acting on it. The ten-minute rule gives you time to decide on something smarter to eat, gives you a few minutes to distract yourself with a positive substitute activity (see "Choosing substitute behaviors" later in the chapter), or allows you the opportunity to figure out what you really want besides food. (I share ways to evaluate your feelings in the moment and how they relate — or don't relate — to food in Table 9-2 later in this chapter.)

Making a gradual transition versus going cold turkey

As you change your mind-set and your eating habits to reduce sugar, you can experiment with two different approaches. One is to work through a gradual transition in which you phase out sugary foods and make selective substitutions over time. The other approach is to quit sugar cold turkey.

Some folks have better success making a gradual transition away from sugar. A slow transition to healthier eating is often easier on the family, too. This is definitely the case if someone in the family is resistant to improving his or her eating habits. (For more on getting your family on board with your efforts to beat sugar, turn to Chapter 11.)

As with most transformations, seeing big changes can take time. For a gradual transition to the low-sugar lifestyle, pick one change from the following list to make each week or two. Soon you'll find that you've transitioned your eating from reactive sugar-grabbing to purposeful, healthy choices.

✔ **Plan ahead by bringing a snack to work instead of grabbing whatever's available in the break room or vending machine.**

✔ **Instead of using bottled sauces and condiments, start substituting additional fruits and vegetables to flavor your everyday foods.** For example, put fruit in your oatmeal, extra veggies on your sandwich, and fresh salsa on your grilled fish.

✔ **Say no to soda!** Make unsweetened tea or mineral water with fresh citrus instead.

✔ **Start cutting back on white-flour starches and start adding more vegetables.** Foods like white breads and pastas, bagels, tortilla chips, and croissants are low in nutrients and fiber and high in calories and carbohydrates. Try replacing white-flour products with whole-grain or non-wheat choices like brown rice pasta, quinoa, or yams.

✔ **Make enough low-sugar dinner to provide leftovers for lunch the next day.** That way you're not at the mercy of trying to find something healthy while eating out.

✔ **If you buy processed or canned foods, look for organic and minimally processed brands without high-fructose corn syrup or artificial sweeteners.**

✔ **Pick a weekend day when you and your family cook everything from scratch.** It's fun, it's quality family time, and you'll have lots of healthy food ready for the rest of the week!

My recommendation for most people is to attempt a gradual transition to a no/low-sugar lifestyle if at all possible. However, some folks do better just going cold turkey — cutting out their sugar intake completely in one fell swoop. If you know yourself well enough to know that the only way for you to break the cycle of sugar addiction is to quit sugar completely, here are some things you can expect:

✔ **Your family may not want to transition with you, and you may face an uproar if their current eating style is disrupted.** You may have to buy and prepare special foods just for you. Hopefully they'll come around eventually.

If you've decided to quit sugar and you find that family members are resistant to switching to healthier eating habits, you may have more success by using the gradual approach with the rest of the family. Making a few healthy substitutions here and there will likely draw little attention, and over the course of a few months you can gradually transition your family to a complete low-sugar lifestyle without them feeling like they've been hoodwinked.

✔ **You'll be tired for the first week or two.** Dreadfully tired. Over the years of addiction, you've likely taught your system to rely on sugar and caffeine for energy, and now you're asking your body to step up and function normally without these substances and without any notice or preparation. Stick with it; it gets better soon!

✔ **Your appetite will change.** Some people report that they're much less hungry after they stop eating sugar. Others report the opposite. Whichever the case is for you, just remember that things will level out in about two weeks, so sit tight and stay on track!

✔ **You'll stop craving most sugar after you've been clean for a week or two, and regular, healthy food (like vegetables) will taste better and be more flavorful to you after you've retrained your taste buds (and your brain) to be accustomed to a normal level of stimulation.**

If quitting sugar cold turkey sounds like the best approach for you, check out Chapter 8 for instructions and advice.

Shopping with purpose

Unless you grow and raise all your own food, mindful grocery shopping is an integral part of staying prepared and purposeful. A simple grocery list that you keep handy (I leave mine out on the kitchen counter) is a very important planning tool. When you see you're close to running out of an item, write it down. Before you go to the grocery store or the farmers' market, think about the next few days of eating. How many protein servings do you need? How much produce? Do you have snacks ready? Write it all down on the list. It sounds simple, but remember that you have to have a plan ready to execute. Otherwise, you won't be prepared and you can easily fall back on reactive, mindless habits. Not planning ahead is one of the things that has kept you stuck in your sugar-loving lifestyle until now.

Here are some other grocery shopping tips to help you succeed in cutting sugar:

✔ **Don't shop when you're hungry.** When your blood sugar is low, you go into survival mode and can lose the ability to make good decisions.

✔ **Focus your food shopping on the outer perimeter of the store — produce, meats and seafood, eggs, and dairy.** Most of your food should come from the perimeter. Most of the processed food that's loaded with sugar and chemicals is located in the center aisles.

✔ **Don't buy tempting junk food "just for the kids" or "just for my spouse."** If you haven't planned well and it's in the house when you're starving, there's going to be trouble. Your family shouldn't be eating that stuff anyway!

✔ **Stick to your list!** Don't take home enticing impulse buys from the checkout counter.

Unraveling Those Overwhelming Sugar Cravings

Sun Tzu, the great military strategist, advised, "Know thyself, know thy enemy." This couldn't be better advice as you work toward freeing yourself from the grip of sugar addiction. You must figure out why you've been fooling yourself all these years, and you must understand why you've fallen victim to the false lure of unhealthy eating.

Though this section isn't intended to feel like it belongs in a psychology book, it's important for you to understand the genesis of your sugar cravings and uncover what you really need instead.

Understanding why cravings occur

In a nutshell, sugar cravings are chemical reactions or learned emotional responses (or sometimes both) that typically originate from one of these common situations or conditions:

- **Abrupt weight loss:** A common condition that triggers a physiological sugar craving is losing weight too quickly (commonly the result of crash dieting). Your body has chemical sensors that trigger an alarm if calorie intake drops too low or if fat storage drops too quickly, and the brain turns on the craving center to replace those calories.

- **Emotional need for serotonin:** *Serotonin* is one of the feel-good hormones that gives you that warm, fuzzy, satisfied (and sometimes sleepy) feeling. If your life doesn't supply you with enough natural happiness (or if you're clinically depressed), your brain seeks out serotonin elsewhere. Sugar, conveniently enough, causes your pancreas to secrete a big spike of insulin to control your blood sugar levels. Insulin eventually triggers the brain to produce serotonin. They don't call sugar a "comfort food" for nothing!

- **Hormonal fluctuations:** Before menstruation, estrogen is low, and as progesterone falls, your endorphin levels are at their lowest. Monthly hormonal fluctuations can explain why many women who experience strong PMS symptoms also have strong sugar cravings — the low endorphin levels cause them to seek out the serotonin burst that a sugar overload can provide.

- **Inadequate nutrition:** If your diet is deficient in certain nutrients, your brain turns on the craving center to try to increase nutrient intake. Your body is programmed to seek out high-calorie (which, in the cave man days, meant *high-nutrient*) foods, so when your body's computer senses a lack of nutrition, it turns on the cravings with full force as a survival mechanism. Check out Table 9-1 for more on nutrient deficiencies.

✔ **Learned behavior to mask loneliness, boredom, or self-deprecation:** As mentioned earlier, sugar equals serotonin. If you're feeling bad, eating sugar can temporarily make you feel better. It's very easy to learn how to substitute unhealthy eating habits for introspection and personal work. When the inner critic starts scolding you, an easy way to quiet the critic is to drug yourself with sugar. The same goes for when you're feeling lonely, bored, or anything else you don't particularly like to feel. Instead of doing the hard personal work that's required to change their ways of thinking and interacting with the world, many people take the easy way out and ignore their problems by zoning out with sugar (or sometimes even worse drugs).

✔ **Stress:** When your body churns out cortisol and other stress hormones all day, you burn up stored carbohydrate (instead of fat) for energy so your brain turns on the craving center to replace that sugar.

Filling the hole: What do you really want?

Abstinence won't keep you off sugar for good. To successfully beat sugar addiction, you must change your relationship with food by finding wisdom and healing at the root of what's incomplete or incongruous in your life.

I always encourage my clients to really dig deep into their alleged desire for sugar. One of my psychology mentors, Anke Nowicki, taught me the life-changing skill of learning to ask myself the right questions to uncover what I was really thinking, wanting, or even blatantly making up. Although introspection and self-discovery are lifetime pursuits, the following sections introduce some basic concepts that may help you become more self-aware right away.

Ask what you really need

When you have an urge to grab something sweet, stop for a moment and answer these questions:

✔ Am I hungry?

✔ Am I tired?

✔ Am I thirsty?

✔ Am I bored?

✔ Am I lonely?

✔ Am I feeling bad about myself or about something else?

✔ Am I overwhelmed or feeling stressed?

Chances are you want something besides sugar. After you identify the real issue, you can start to find ways to satisfy what you really need instead of medicating yourself with sugar.

Look at the circumstances that preceded the craving

People are creatures of habit. If you start to look for patterns in your cravings for sugar, you'll probably notice that when certain things happen, your brain turns on the craving center. Next time you have an unhealthy craving, look at the circumstances that preceded it. Here are some situations that commonly precede a sugar craving:

✔ When you don't sleep well

✔ When you feel overwhelmed at work

✔ When you feel unloved by your spouse

✔ When you feel out of control about a family situation

✔ When you haven't eaten for a few hours

✔ When you haven't had enough water

✔ After you've eaten too many carbs and not enough protein and fat

✔ When you're worried or anxious about something

✔ After you've eaten too much

✔ When you can't find anything interesting to think about or to create

✔ When you think about a yummy treat that's in the pantry

✔ When you feel like you want to reward yourself

If you notice a consistent pattern of cravings after one or more of these situations, change or attend to the situation or condition that precedes the craving. One of the easiest ways to beat sugar cravings is to avoid or fix the situations that trigger them in the first place. Don't play in traffic!

Letting your craving tell you what's missing from your nutrition

Cravings can often be a signal from your body that you're missing some important nutrients. Table 9-1 shows some possible correlations.

Table 9-1	Nutritional Deficiencies That Can Cause Cravings	
If You Crave or Have This	**You May Be Deficient In**	**Get What You Need from These Foods**
Chocolate	Magnesium	Bran, raw nuts and seeds, legumes, spinach
Toasted bread	Nitrogen	High protein foods (fish, meat, eggs)
Fatty or oily foods	Calcium	Dark greens (spinach, mustard, turnip, kale), broccoli, cheese, yogurt
Chewing ice	Iron	Meat, poultry, seaweed, greens, raisins
Burned food	Carbon	Fresh fruits and vegetables
Carbonated drinks	Calcium	Dark greens (spinach, mustard, turnip, kale), broccoli, cheese, yogurt
Salty foods	Chloride	Fish, sea salt, goat milk
Acid foods	Magnesium	Bran, raw nuts and seeds, legumes, spinach
Preference for liquids instead of solid food	Water	Flavor with fresh citrus if you like
Avoidance of liquids in preference of solid foods instead	Water	You've been dehydrated for so long that your thirst center has melded with your hunger center; drink small amounts (4 to 6 ounces) of water every one to two hours throughout the day
Premenstrual cravings	Zinc	Red meats, oysters, root vegetables
Ravenous appetite (without having gone too long without food)	Silicon	Bananas, green beans, oats, whole grains; avoid white "enriched" flour
	Tryptophan	Dairy, lamb, turkey
	Tyrosine	L-tyrosine supplement, orange and red vegetables and fruits
	Dietary fat	Fish oil, olive oil, cheese
Lack of appetite	B vitamins	Meats, organ meats, seeds and legumes, grains
Sweets	Chromium	Multivitamin/mineral supplement, broccoli, grapes, mushrooms, whole grains
	Magnesium	Bran, raw nuts and seeds, legumes, spinach

Managing Cravings

Even after you've started to change your thinking, your habits, and your food content, your sugar cravings won't disappear overnight. Unlearning old habits and old ways of thinking is a process, and while you work on improving your ways of eating and thinking, you're bound to experience occasional sugar cravings. This section talks about things you can do to minimize these cravings, identifies common triggers, and walks you through the exact steps of what to do when a craving strikes.

Timing your meals properly

To keep your blood sugar levels stable and ward off emergency cravings for energy, it's important to eat often. A good rule of thumb is to eat a combination of protein and carbohydrates every three to four hours. If you go longer than that without eating, your body goes into "starvation emergency" mode and starts holding on to its fat stores and cranking up the appetite center. By eating small amounts of quality food every few hours, your blood sugar levels stay nice and even all day, and your body happily uses fat as its preferred energy source for your activities.

Another good reason to eat often enough is that the amino acids from protein only survive for a few hours after digestion. If you go longer than that without eating a protein source, your body begins to break down muscle tissue (and organs!) in a process called *catabolism* to replenish the missing amino acids. Any eating habits that cause loss of muscle tissue lower your metabolism.

Following smart nutrition practices

In addition to meal timing, you can use the following nutrition practices to help ward off cravings. If you'd like to dive deeper into these principles, you can find a more detailed look at nutrition in Chapter 5.

- **Drink enough water.** Often, people who are chronically dehydrated lose their sensation of thirst. The thirst center in the brain then melds with the hunger center, so many folks who are unknowingly dehydrated get a food craving when what they really need is water. Dehydration also increases fatigue and decreases mental alertness.

- **Avoid artificial sweeteners.** Aspartame (NutraSweet) is a chemical that's harmful to your brain, and some studies show that it increases appetite. Regularly over-stimulating the taste centers of the brain with artificial sweeteners increases the desire for that extra-sweet taste. If you absolutely must flavor your beverages, use stevia root powder instead of sugar or chemicals.

✔ **Eat enough during the day.** Big drops in your blood sugar level lead to big cravings for sugar and carbs to bring it back up. Sometimes, the late-night cravings are a signal that you haven't eaten enough earlier in the day, and your body is looking to make up those extra calories.

✔ **Eat lots of vegetables.** Here are three main reasons that snacking on vegetables can help stave off sugar cravings:

- Vegetables are high in nutrients and low in calories. Remember that a deficiency in certain nutrients can turn on the craving center.

- The crunch factor that many vegetables possess gives you a satisfying chewing experience and pleasurable mouth feel. Many sugar addicts (and smoking addicts, too) have reported to me that the mouth feel is one of the main reasons they seek out snacking or smoking, so crunchy vegetables can serve as a much healthier option to fill that desire.

- The fiber in vegetables helps you feel full. Research shows that your stomach gets accustomed to a particular volume of food, so you often won't feel satisfied until you've ingested a particular amount of food, regardless of its calorie content. Eating lots of high-volume, low-calorie vegetables helps you feel full without going overboard on the calories.

✔ **Plan ahead.** Remember that most of the convenience food that's available quickly isn't very healthy. Before you leave the house (or even the night before), be sure to plan your eating for the day. Either bring your low-sugar options with you or have a plan in place for what and where you'll eat throughout the day.

Identifying triggers

Triggers are events or situations to which people react. Often in the case of the sugar addict, those reactions are habits that are both learned and chemically induced. To consciously change your reactions to triggers, you must first identify that you're reacting to a situation.

Here's a new drill for you to practice:

1. **Every time you have a craving, stop and ask yourself what you're reacting to.**

   Is it hunger? A stressful event? An inconsiderate spouse? Thirst? Loneliness?

2. **Take a moment to figure out what you really want (it's not sugar).**

3. **Ask yourself whether eating sugar is going to give you what you really want.**

   My guess is no. . . .

Use the examples in Table 9-2 to help get you started with this self-questioning habit.

Table 9-2	Adding a Reality Check to Your Triggers	
What Happened	*What I Want*	*Reality Check*
I have stressful deadlines at work.	To feel confident that I will get everything done in time	Will eating sugar give me that confidence?
I feel hopeless.	Hope	Will eating sugar give me hope?
I'm lonely.	Companionship	Will eating sugar give me companionship?
I feel fat or unattractive.	To feel better about myself	Will eating sugar make me feel better about myself?
Something my partner said or did made me feel unhappy or stressed.	To feel reassured and reconnected to my partner	Will eating sugar give me that connection?
I'm bored.	Something engaging for my mind	Will eating sugar give me something interesting to do?
I feel like my life is out of control.	Peace and personal power	Will eating sugar give me peace and power?

Choosing substitute behaviors

Another technique you can use to stay away from sweets is to find a substitute activity to engage in whenever you have a sugar craving. I've found that it's important for people to find activities that they enjoy and that they find meaningful. Doing something good for someone else is a great way to get your mind off sugar! Here's a list of some suggestions:

- Take a walk.
- Ride your bike.

- ✔ Grab a digital camera or your cellphone and go look for interesting or artistic pictures to take.

- ✔ Make a list of things to talk about with your partner, therapist, or best friend.

- ✔ Read something interesting.

- ✔ Play with your pet. If you don't have a pet, go to a shelter and give some love to one of the animals there.

- ✔ Phone a friend or family member to catch up.

- ✔ Look up a long-lost friend on Facebook and say hi.

- ✔ Write an apology letter to someone you've wronged.

- ✔ Find a new charity you like and send a donation.

- ✔ If you have a partner, write a love note.

- ✔ Visit someone in the hospital or in hospice.

- ✔ Do a Sudoku puzzle or play chess or Scrabble on the computer — keep your brain occupied!

- ✔ Do some crunches or jumping jacks.

- ✔ Update your bucket list.

- ✔ Pick something in the house that needs to be fixed or cleaned and attend to it.

- ✔ Look up a subject that interests you and learn something new about it.

- ✔ Make a list of movies you want to see or books you want to read.

Share your own favorite positive behavior substitutions and read about what others are doing on our discussion group at www.BeatingSugar Addiction.com.

Acting when a craving strikes

In spite of your best efforts to prevent sugar cravings, you're likely to find yourself facing one eventually. Knowing a few defensive maneuvers helps ensure that you get past the craving without totally derailing your low-sugar plan — although if you do fall off the wagon, the next section helps you get back on. This section is, in my humble opinion, one of the most valuable parts of this entire book — a step-by-step guide of exactly what to do when a sugar craving strikes!

When a craving strikes, follow these steps:

1. **Drink a cold glass of distilled water or citrus-flavored mineral water.**

2. **Identify what triggered the craving (refer to the "Identifying triggers" section earlier in the chapter).**

   Don't allow yourself to have the treat until you come up with the answer.

3. **Make a conscious decision to eat or not eat the sweet.**

   Remember, you're the boss of your behavior. No one makes you do anything. If you decide to eat some sugar, you must own it and do it on purpose — don't make any excuses or point any fingers!

If you decide *not* to eat something sweet, choose one or more of these rewards:

✔ Give yourself a (healthy) personal reward! Draw a smiley face on the calendar, put a dollar in the cookie jar (because you don't keep cookies in the house anymore), or take yourself to the movies.

✔ Tell someone! Call or e-mail a friend, write a blog post or a Facebook update, and so on.

✔ Choose a positive substitute activity if you want (see the preceding section).

If you decide to eat something sweet, stick to these rules:

✔ You must abide by the ten-minute rule — you have to wait ten minutes before you eat a sugary treat. If you still want it after ten minutes, go ahead.

✔ Put the amount you'll eat on a plate first — no eating from packages or serving dishes.

✔ Try a substitute sweet fix:

   • Decaf green tea, or, if you're an Exhausted Addict (see Chapter 2), licorice tea to help restore adrenal function

   • A small portion of a low-glycemic fruit like cherries, apple, or plum

   • A tic tac or Altoid mint

   • Ice water sweetened with stevia

   • A couple squares of sugar-free chocolate

Coping with Falling Off the Wagon

No one is perfect, and no one eats perfectly all the time. The good news is you don't have to! The key to long-term success is to learn how to make good decisions on a regular basis and not to get derailed just because you've had a less-than-mindful day.

Starting with forgiveness

Mindful eating is a process, a practice that requires, well, practice! You won't be perfect right off the bat. Being mindful about what you eat doesn't mean being neurotic, obsessive, or fearful about food. To heal sugar addiction (or addiction of any type), you have to heal the emotional brain that you've taught, unknowingly, to crave something to medicate yourself. It's not easy; you're going to have to do some work to stay mindful and build new, healthy habits.

If you make a bad decision or even if you have a whole day of horrible eating, recognize what you did (no excuses), then forgive yourself, with the intention that you'll do better next time. You're not a failure, a freak, or a hopeless screw-up. Due to biology, society, and your past habits and behaviors, you've become an addict and you need help. It takes time and practice to undo all that past learning. Cut yourself some slack — no one's behavior is perfect 100 percent of the time.

There's a big difference between recognizing a mistake and judging yourself. Scolding yourself only worsens your self-negativity and triggers the emotional insecurities that drive the desire for comfort food in the first place.

Dealing with the inner critic

If you're like most who struggle with addictive personalities, you probably have a well-developed inner critic — the voice continually jabbering away at you, looking for anything to find fault with. It magnifies small failings into giant ones, chastises you over and over for things long past, ignores the true context, and doesn't credit you for any of your successes. Sound familiar?

What does the inner critic want? It wants to be right. It wants to find evidence to support the same old stories it always tells you. Imagine your inner critic as an obnoxious person at the office who sits around and does nothing except accusingly point at people and say, "See? See, I told you _____!"

Don't pay any attention to this crazy person. It has nothing positive to offer you and is totally out of touch with the facts. It's just desperately trying to be right, because that's its only job description. If it can't prove it's right, it gets fired. That's right, you can fire your inner critic if you want to! All you have to do is listen objectively to the story or the "evidence" and determine if it's really true.

Here's an example of questioning the inner critic's "evidence": After a bad food choice, your inner critic shouts, "See? I told you how stupid you are; now you've ruined everything!" Is this true? Are you stupid because you made a bad decision? Have you really "ruined everything"? Certainly not! Successfully beating sugar is a series of ongoing decisions, and you blew one of them. Big deal. You'll get it right next time; you don't have to start all over like this character is telling you.

After a few times that the inner critic comes to you with evidence that you determine isn't true, you can fire it easily and deservedly.

A great book for learning to ask the right "Is it true?" questions is Byron Katie's *Loving What Is: Four Questions That Can Change Your Life*. If you have a strong inner critic and you haven't read it, I strongly suggest that you do.

Getting back on track: Three easy steps

Because success with low-sugar eating is an ongoing series of small decisions, when you make a bad decision it's important to be able to get back to making smart ones right away. Follow these three easy steps and you'll be right back on the wagon:

1. **State what you did without judging, exaggerating, or catastrophizing.**

   Just the facts, ma'am. Examples might be, "I ate a sweet roll for a snack," or "I ate a bag of M&Ms."

2. **State why you did it.**

   This one is hard because you have to look past any story that you told yourself and reveal the truth. The story may be, "I didn't have time to eat something healthy." The real truth is, "I was hungry, and I didn't bring any good food with me, and I decided I would rather eat the sweet roll than stay hungry."

3. **State what you intend to do next time.**

   "Tomorrow I will bring a healthy snack to work."

Chapter 10

Navigating the Minefields of Eating Out and Special Occasions

· ·

· ·

*E*ven when you get your day-to-day eating under control at home and at work, eating well when you're out at restaurants or celebrating special occasions can still be a daunting challenge. Restaurant menus are filled with scrumptious creations that are often packed with fat and sugar, and the holiday season lures people into a sense of abandon when it comes to the endless amounts of delicious, high-sugar goodies that are constantly available. On top of those, add the occasional dinner party, birthday, or other celebration, and you may find that a third of your meals (or more) over the course of a year are "abnormal" — which is code for "I ate way too much food, and most of it was junk."

In this chapter, I give you strategies for making smart choices at restaurants and tips for eating out without pigging out. I discuss ways for you to eat reasonably during the holidays and other special events, so you can still enjoy yourself while sticking to your low-sugar or no-sugar goals.

Eating Out Successfully

Mindfulness and planning are very important to prevent the act of eating out from turning into a nutritional disaster. Restaurants serve up enticing appetizer and entree concoctions topped with sauces loaded with fat and sugar, and they deliver portions large enough for a whole family. Then they tease you with a delightful dessert menu that would drive any pastry lover mad with envy. If you place your orders impulsively, based solely on what sounds good or looks good, you'll derail your sugar-busting food plan before you know what happened. The key to long-term dietary success is making sure you're always in control.

Watching portion sizes

When eating out at a restaurant, it's safe to assume that you're getting two or three servings on your plate (see Chapter 5 for information on portions). Here are three tips to keep from overeating at restaurants:

- ✔ **Pay attention to how much you eat, how fast you eat, and whether you really need any more food in your stomach.** See Chapter 8 for more advice on mindfulness and proactive eating.

- ✔ **Eat vegetables first, then protein.** After that, decide whether you really want (or need) any of the extra starch (rice, pasta, bread, and so on) on your plate.

- ✔ **When you place your order, ask the server to bring a takeout container with your meal.** When it arrives, put half of what's on the plate into your takeout container before you even start eating. You'll never miss the other half, and you can enjoy it the next day.

Allocating alcohol and dessert

If you don't eat out very often, it's okay to make the experience special. Don't put yourself in food jail on your birthday or anniversary — go ahead and indulge in something that you ordinarily wouldn't eat. Just don't go so far overboard that you later wish you hadn't done it. I typically suggest that when you eat out for a special occasion, have one drink and choose between an appetizer and half a dessert. And for the record, you're not required to eat all of whatever you choose!

If you eat out several times per week, the restaurant experience is no longer special; it's just a method of feeding yourself. Treat your day-to-day restaurant meals just like you would any other — minding your sugar content, portions, protein/carb ratios, and other standard nutrition variables that you've now learned to pay attention to. Don't get dazzled by the location — *what* you eat is much more important than *where* you eat it.

Staying mindful

When you're eating out at a restaurant or at a party, chances are that everyone's focus is on the conversation instead of the food, so be careful not to use external cues (like an empty plate) as the only signals for when you've had enough to eat. Frequently turn your attention inward and pay attention to what you're doing and how you're feeling. Ask yourself questions like

> ✔ Am I eating too fast or not chewing thoroughly?
>
> ✔ Do I really need more food or could I stop eating right now?
>
> ✔ How does my stomach feel?
>
> ✔ How much have I had to drink?
>
> ✔ When is the last time I really tasted what I'm eating?

When looking over the menu, be sure that all the basic nutrition bases are covered in your decisions: Double-check that you have vegetables and protein on your plate, that your choice is low-sugar, and that your portions are reasonable. Smart decisions when ordering make it easier to temper your behavior while eating. See Chapter 5 for an overview of nutrition basics and for assistance with choosing low-glycemic carbohydrates.

Choosing best bet basics

If you're worried about sugar content, calories, or other dietary considerations when eating out (and you should at least be thinking about these), you can't go wrong with vegetables and lean protein. Endless varieties of delicious meals are available that are heavy on veggies and protein and low on sugar, starches, and sauces. When in doubt, your best bet basics are meals with a protein source (chicken, fish, lamb, duck, and so on) and a pile of vegetables without too much stuff on them. Often, a salad of organic mixed greens topped with salmon, shrimp, or meat tossed in the house's specialty vinaigrette can be one of the most delightful dishes on the menu, not to mention a healthy alternative to some of the many calorie-and-sugar-laden entrees available.

If you're not sure how something on the menu is prepared, don't be afraid to ask. Most kitchens are happy to make you a version of a dish without the sauce or to come up with a sugar-free alternative. Having worked in restaurant kitchens myself, I can say from personal experience that sometimes it's a nice change for the cook to be able to use some creativity and make something different from the usual.

Navigating Social Eating

Staying on track while eating in social situations — dinner parties, date nights, wedding receptions, and similar events — can be challenging, to say the least. Typically, the fare served by caterers and restaurants is much higher in sugar, fat, calories, and portion size than what you'd ordinarily eat, and you'll likely be focused on everything except what (and how) you're eating. Being aware of your food intake while fully participating in all the social interaction takes some practice, but by utilizing a few of the basic skills in the following sections, you should be able to stay proactive with your food and still have a great time!

Preventing common mistakes

A handful of social situations often crop up that can destroy your nutrition plan if you're not careful. If you can avoid these common pitfalls, you'll have a much easier time keeping the event from turning into an eating disaster:

✔ **Eating everything you're given:** Many events have a constant flow of food coming at you from all directions, much of it carbohydrates. News flash — you don't have to eat everything that someone hands you. Choose your snacks wisely.

✔ **Playing the "I'll have some if you have some" game:** People often look toward another's behavior to give them permission to eat dessert or junk food. Just because your friend wants some dessert doesn't mean you're obligated to eat some too. It's not rude for one person not to eat something that others are eating, so don't fall into the social trap of using what others do as an excuse not to make your own decisions.

✔ **Staying near the food all night:** People love to congregate in the kitchen or near the buffet line, but conversations don't have to stay there all night. You can be the one who invites people to move to a different area by saying something like, "Let's move away from these cookies before I eat them all." You may even be helping out some other folks who may be trying to clean up their eating too. If you stand and talk next to the brownie plate all night, you're just asking for trouble!

Being prepared

If you're headed to a place or an event where you know that the food will be unhealthy, plan ahead and arrive having already eaten a healthy, sugar-free meal. If you show up hungry and all that's available is junk food, you'll probably succumb to your hunger and cravings before you can get something better to eat later on.

If you're not able to eat a full, healthy meal before a social dining event, at least make sure that you eat often enough throughout the day so that you don't arrive with a hungry belly. Walking into a room filled with tempting junk food when you haven't eaten for six or seven hours is a disaster waiting to happen. Plan ahead!

Creating balance

As discussed in Chapter 8, beware of becoming obsessive or neurotic about food. If you're at a special event and you spend all your time and energy being super-strict about what you eat, you may find that you feel disappointed even though you ate well, because you've missed out on what was supposed to be important.

I've heard clients talk about an event or party with fear in their voice, simply because they knew desserts would be there. If you have that attitude, you'll most likely have a miserable time no matter what the event because you'll be so afraid you may succumb to the allure of sugar that you won't be able to relax and enjoy yourself. This is both sad and unhealthy. Empower yourself, and always remember that you're the one who makes every single decision about your actions and your attitude.

One of the keys to creating balance with eating is that you must feel good about doing it. If having desserts and treats in moderation feels like punishment, then you'll feel like it's dieting instead of normal eating, and you won't likely maintain the moderate approach for long. See Chapter 9 for tips on the important concept of creating a "new normal."

I encourage you to lighten up and allow yourself to eat a reasonable amount of junk food at a special event. Just promise to do it on purpose, not unconsciously, and to stay mindful about what you choose to do — no "brain off" gluttony allowed! Limit your portions of bad food to a few bites, and eat slowly. If you find that you're not enjoying what you're eating, don't finish it.

Reprogramming an all-or-nothing attitude about sweets

An all-or-nothing attitude toward food is one of the most dangerous traps for the sugar addict. If you try to remain on an overly restrictive eating plan, you'll eventually give in to your cravings because hardly anyone can stay on an "absolutely none" plan for very long. After you give in to your old habits, the all-or-nothing mind-set will swing you to the other end of the spectrum, and you'll overindulge in a way that would embarrass a hedonistic Roman emperor.

The problem with having an all-or-nothing mentality is that you treat your improved eating plan as a temporary restriction, not as a new way of eating or thinking about food. Reprogramming the all-or-nothing attitude allows you to enjoy all foods in your diet, even some dessert, just not with complete abandon. Your goal with improved eating habits should be to create a "new normal" so that you never feel like you're on a diet or a restricted eating plan (see Chapter 9).

A party, an event, or a holiday is *not* the last time you'll have the opportunity to eat your favorite junk foods. When you have a new normal, you don't follow a strict diet, so you aren't deprived of these foods forever. When you decide to indulge in a treat, have a few bites, and then call it quits. You don't have to eat a lifetime of sugar in one night!

Surviving Vacations and Special Occasions

Throughout the course of a year, you'll experience stretches of time where sugar and junk food are plentiful, like vacations and holidays. The tips in the following sections can help you keep tabs on your sugar intake while still enjoying some treats in moderation during these times. These tips guide you through making the best choices out of whatever food is available to help you stay on track.

Vacations

When you're on vacation, throwing temperance to the wind is easy, especially if you're in a situation where high-sugar food is omnipresent, like a cruise ship or a festival. Cutting loose and lightening up on what you allow yourself to eat while on vacation is okay, but if you pull out all the stops and go overboard, you can do a lot of damage in a short period of time.

Vacation should be a time for you to relax, get out of your normal routine, spend some quality time with loved ones, and soak up some special life experiences. Some indulgent cuisine can be part of that, but the focus of your vacation shouldn't be stuffing yourself with as many carbohydrates as you can find. Keep your focus on decompressing and on enjoying great experiences, not on seeing how much you can devour from the dessert bar before you make yourself sick.

Holidays

It amazes me how many people completely shut off any sensibility or moderation around food during holidays. When they give themselves permission to indulge in some holiday sweets, an all-or-nothing mentality takes over, and they go completely overboard, gobbling down every single sugar-filled treat they can lay their hands on — usually with the promise that at the beginning of the new year they'll start their diet, get back to the gym, or whatever other promise they make to themselves every year. It's almost like they've entered a contest in their minds, trying to win the award for who can cram the most sugar into themselves before New Year's.

I encourage you to enjoy some goodies during holiday times, but you need to do so in a reasonable fashion. If you're at a holiday party with a table loaded with desserts as far as the eye can see, pick three things and have two bites of each one. That way you'll get to enjoy three desserts without overloading yourself with sugar.

During the holidays, you don't need to splurge at every meal of every day. The holiday season isn't a pass to eat foolishly for weeks! Do some planning in advance and look for times when it will be easy for you to put together a healthy meal. Be on the lookout for situations in which you'll want to overindulge, and be judicious about which ones you allow to become major deviations from your healthy, low-sugar lifestyle. Pick your battles and make conscious, sensible decisions about when you have a treat and how much of it you eat.

During the holiday season, don't lose sight of the big picture of a healthy nutrition plan — things like vegetables, protein, water, and portion control. Consider junk food as extra, not as a substitute for real food. Be sure to apportion your treat before you start eating so you can keep the amount of sugar you consume in check. You don't have to eat *all* the cookies to enjoy them!

Birthdays and other special occasions

The fact that you're celebrating a special occasion such as a birthday or an anniversary doesn't mean that you must eat foolishly. Don't feel obligated to eat dessert or drink too much to get the most out of your celebration. Focus on the special people around you instead of the junk food that's available.

Past conditioning may have led you to believe that it's okay to eat all bad foods on special occasions. This unhealthy mind-set reinforces sugar as a reward or as a necessary part of special times.

A good strategy to help you stay sugar-free during special occasions is to distinguish between tummy hungry and yummy hungry. *Tummy hungry* is when you want to eat because you listen to the cues that your body gives you, and you're actually hungry. *Yummy hungry* is when you want to eat because you see something that looks enticing. Stay mindful by paying attention to what your body tells you, and don't allow your eyes to dictate your mouth's behavior. The next time you get a craving to eat something, pause for a moment to assess whether you're truly tummy hungry or just piqued by a yummy hungry prospect.

Chapter 11

Getting a Boost from Your Support System

- -

In This Chapter

▶ Dealing with other people's negativity

▶ Building a support system among family, friends, and co-workers

▶ Using support groups and Internet forums to stay on track

▶ Getting professional help

- -

*A*s you begin your quest to beat sugar addiction and lead a healthier lifestyle, building a support system around you encourages you and helps hold you accountable. A support system also gives you a close ring of people with whom you can share both your triumphs and your setbacks.

In this chapter, I share some ideas for building a reliable support system — who to include, who not to include, and how to be prepared for the naysayers and saboteurs you'll encounter. I give you some tips for bringing your family on board and lay out some options for support groups that you may not have thought of. Lastly, I present some advice for choosing the right professional help when you need it.

Countering the "War on Food" Mentality

When it comes to food, not following the herd can be challenging. If you announce to your friends and family that you've decided to overcome your addiction to sugar, be prepared for some unexpected reactions. Though some people will congratulate you and wish you the best, others will react as if you're declaring war on their own favorite foods. Be prepared for people who you thought were your friends to make fun of you, to tell you you're crazy, or to harrumph about how you'll never be able to sustain the low-sugar lifestyle. Do your best to ignore these people, and let them have their own issues; it's not your mission to gather approval from every person you know.

Brenner FIT 5-4-3-2-1-0 program

The health risks associated with childhood obesity are regularly discussed, but kids' emotional risks are sometimes forgotten. Overweight children are often teased at school, on the playground, and even at home. They look different from other children and know it, but they can't make the changes they need to make on their own.

The Brenner Children's Hospital of Wake Forest Baptist Medical Center has instituted a program to help combat the epidemic of childhood obesity. Families work with a team that includes a doctor, a family counselor, a dietitian, an exercise specialist, and a social worker, with the goal of helping the entire family change its lifestyle.

The program doesn't put families on restrictive diets or ban all sweets, because losing weight shouldn't be a punishment. The plan does adjust the family's diet, implement regular physical activity, and teach the family how to plan a weekly menu and buy healthy foods on a tight budget.

The crux of the Brenner FIT (families in training) program is the 5-4-3-2-1-0 system. Even without a team of professionals to advise and assist you, you can apply the following tenets to your own family's routine to reap the plan's benefits:

5 Eat five servings of fruits and vegetables each day.

4 Eat together as a family at least four times a week.

3 Eat three healthy meals a day — no skipping meals, especially breakfast.

2 Limit screen time (computer, TV, and video games) to less than two hours a day.

1 Aim for one hour of physical activity each day.

0 Reduce the number of sugar-sweetened drinks like sodas and juice to zero.

Try gradually implementing these changes into your family's lifestyle, and watch your waistlines shrink and your health skyrocket!

Consult Chapter 9 for tips on gradually introducing healthier foods into your household.

When you're met with skepticism, don't fall victim to other people's fears and negativity. Keep in mind that you're not completely banning sugar from your life; you're just changing the way you usually do things and making better decisions across the board.

Eating better isn't a big hairy monster that you're required to battle at every meal. Taking better care of yourself is merely a series of ongoing smart decisions that lead you where you want to go, both physically and emotionally. Focus on consistency, not on waging war against food. Consult Chapter 9 for tips on creating a new, healthy "normal."

Bringing Your Family on Board

By trying to get your family to cooperate in your endeavors to eat better, you may end up with a loving circle of family support or you may end up completely disappointed. It's usually one or the other. Changing your own diet and habits often means some changes for the rest of the family too, and family members who are set in their ways don't always accept those changes painlessly or with open minds.

You want the best for your family, but don't try to save the world all at once. Focus on your own choices and behaviors first, and perhaps your good examples (and better mood!) will start to rub off on other members of your household. Remember that you can't change other people; you can only change yourself.

Enlisting Friends and Co-workers

Confiding in a small group of friends who know you well can strengthen your support system. However, involving the right friends is important because you won't receive the right kind of support from everyone you know. The following sections explain how to involve the right people and how to avoid those who will drag you down.

Supporters

The ideal support partners are friends who truly support your goals to free yourself from the grip of sugar and to lead a healthier life that's under control. Your closest friends may not necessarily be the best folks for you to look to for support because they may not be in your shoes and may not understand what the big deal is all about.

You'll probably receive the best support and accountability from friends who are looking to improve their own eating habits and lifestyles, even if they're not your closest friends. Your best ally may turn out to be someone you barely know! Look for people in your circle who are already living the lifestyle you aspire to. They can serve as great role models and wonderful sources of advice and encouragement.

Naysayers

Regardless of how close you feel to your friends and family members, I guarantee that some of them will unknowingly act as naysayers and saboteurs, so be emotionally ready for this to happen. You'll have friends or co-workers who may make fun of you for your food choices at restaurants, or your spouse may bring home an ice cream cake the day after you have a tearful conversation about how out of control you feel your life is.

Try to keep in mind that these people are (hopefully) not being mean or insensitive on purpose; they just don't understand how hard making life changes can be. They probably haven't considered making any improvements for themselves or just don't understand what you're going through because they've never tried to overcome any type of addiction.

Whatever the reason for their behavior, try not to hold it against them. People who aren't interested in adopting healthy behaviors themselves often engage in negative talk about yours or downplay the importance of the changes you're trying to make. Don't let it discourage you!

Don't bother talking about dietary stuff or exercise with naysayers — they're just not interested and they'll only bring you down. You have plenty of other things to talk about, so reserve discussions about your personal goals and progress for supportive people who are interested in hearing about your journey.

Devil's advocates

Sometimes your best friends can also be your worst temptations. If you have a friend with whom you often share scripted behavior, like having dessert together every time you go out to lunch somewhere, don't be surprised if she intentionally tempts you with food choices that you're trying to stay away from.

Don't let a distorted sense of loyalty dictate your behavior! Your friend doesn't need you to eat junk food to enjoy your time together, and you haven't abandoned your friend if you decide not to partake in sugary treats that the two of you have historically shared.

Let your would-be devil's advocate know that you're happy with the dietary changes you're making and that you feel great when you don't eat sugar. If your friends and family know that you're happy with the changes you're making, that's what should matter to them.

Evangelists

After your friends and co-workers hear about your quest to kick the sugar habit, you may find that one of them latches on to you and evangelizes non-stop about a particular diet or supplement that has worked miracles for her, or a friend of hers, or her brother-in-law's plumber's wife. Though this person may genuinely have your best interest at heart, she may also be involved in a multilevel marketing supplement company and may be trying to reel you in.

In my experience, evangelists are unable to carry on a conversation without stuffing your ears full of great tales of their miracle thingy. Politely take their brochures or write down the book title or website they're espousing, and say, "I'll check it out, thanks." If the evangelist persists at future encounters, let her know that you appreciate her help and input but that you have a system that's working great right now, and you don't want to screw it up by trying to take on too much.

Finding a Support Group

Collaborating with other people with similar goals and experiences can be a helpful way to share pitfalls and celebrations, especially if they're in similar circumstances. Sometimes, staying on track is easier if you're part of a team on which everyone has the same goal. Hearing others' stories can help validate your own experiences, and sharing your own experiences and advice can help others. When it comes to support groups, the whole is definitely greater than the individual parts.

Getting involved with a local support group

Getting involved in a group therapy session can be an easy way to build a team of support around you. Support groups for various eating issues abound, or you could even start your own! Here are some tips for finding a group to visit:

- Ask a therapist or counselor to recommend a local support group that's appropriate for you.
- Peruse church or temple bulletin boards for notifications of group meetings.

✔ Search www.craigslist.org, http://groups.psychologytoday.com, and http://group-therapy.meetup.com for support groups in your area.

✔ Visit your local Weight Watchers chapter to see whether it offers (or can recommend) additional support group meetings.

If a more nationally organized structure appeals to you, consider finding a local chapter of Overeaters Anonymous or the Eating Disorders Coalition if you feel like those types of groups may be appropriate for you.

Investigating Internet forums

Internet discussion groups are another option for finding advice and motivation. Peers and professionals from all over the world can share stories, struggles, and advice. Internet forums can be great places to obtain general support and encouragement, especially if you're struggling with setbacks. They also afford you a wonderful opportunity to give back to the community by being there for others when they need the same.

Unfortunately, Internet forums have a downside, too. The anonymous nature of the Internet makes it easy for people to post angry or downright offensive comments on group discussion boards. You may also run into evangelists of particular diets or products who are critical of all other diets and products, so be prepared to weed through a lot of negative postings. You'll also encounter a lot of salespeople for particular products.

Seeking Help from a Professional When You Need It

Overhauling a lifetime of destructive food habits can be a daunting task, especially when you also have a lot of other issues with work and family on your plate. Finding a professional therapist or counselor who has helped hundreds of people in your shoes is a smart way to propel your personal growth to a new level, especially if you're struggling with some deep emotional issues like depression, self-criticism, or hopelessness.

One of the things I consistently hear from clients is, "I know what to do; I just can't seem to do it." Because doing is indeed much harder than knowing, receiving some guidance from a professional can help you develop some strategies and tricks to implement the healthy changes that you're having difficulty making on your own.

Nutrition counselors

If you have a challenging health condition like polycystic ovarian syndrome (PCOS), diabetes, kidney disease, or food allergies, I suggest that you find a registered dietitian or qualified nutrition counselor who has experience with that particular condition to assist you with your dietary journey.

Not all nutrition professionals with letters after their names are well educated or well qualified. During your first nutrition counseling appointment, if your counselor hands you a photocopy of the food pyramid or stares blankly at you when you mention probiotic supplements or whey protein, find a different counselor who's more educated in current evidence-based nutrition science.

Consider asking your chiropractor, massage therapist, and/or fitness trainer to recommend a qualified, well-rounded nutrition counselor with whom their clients have had good success.

Psychotherapists

Whether you call yours a counselor, therapist, shrink, guru, spiritual leader, life coach, or psychologist, there's no substitute for having a trained professional help you delve into the how's and why's of your behavior, emotions, and beliefs. Finding an experienced therapist to help guide you through the introspection process is time and money well spent!

Finding a therapist who's a good fit for you may take some time and experimentation. This field has many different approaches and personalities, so be prepared to try out several practitioners until you find one who feels right.

Ask for recommendations from your friends, family, and members of your support team. If that yields no results, you can find local practitioners to interview from www.goodtherapy.org or http://locator.apa.org.

Finding a professional who's good is much more important than finding one who's convenient. Selecting a therapist just because his office is on your way home probably won't yield the best match for you. Doing your own personal work is important, life-changing stuff, so treat it accordingly!

Before booking your first session, talk to the therapist on the phone and get answers to questions like:

- ✔ How many years have you been practicing, and what are your credentials?
- ✔ What are your areas of expertise?
- ✔ Do you have experience with issues like mine?
- ✔ Have you ever been in therapy yourself? You probably shouldn't get into therapy with someone who hasn't done his own work. Seeing a therapist who hasn't done his own therapy is like hiring a personal trainer who doesn't work out or a financial advisor who can't save any money.

While you're on the phone, don't forget to double-check fees, cancellation policies, and insurance details.

Use the list of complementary medicine options in Chapter 7 to give you some ideas for additional professionals who may also be a good fit in your support system.

Chapter 12

Sugar-Busting Moves: Incorporating Exercise

. . . .

. . . .

*P*eople often report a lifetime of frustration with exercise. Even if you can find the time, motivation, and energy to make exercise a regular part of your week, it's easy to get confused by all the conflicting exercise advice that gets thrown at you from magazines, exercise evangelists, misinformed-but-well-intentioned bloggers, and TV gurus.

Adequate and appropriate exercise is a vital component of long-term health, and it's especially important for the sugar addict who wants to lose weight and stay craving-free. My goal in this chapter is to explain the effects that a proper exercise program can have on your body and to lay out the key elements of constructing a successful exercise plan.

Instead of making promises to yourself to start hitting the treadmill yet again, I urge you to take the time to read through this chapter in detail so you can understand the kind of workouts that you need to do. I explain the effectiveness and the proper structure of basic strength training and cardiovascular workouts, so you'll have an efficient, effective system of exercise to help you slim down, get in shape, and stay away from sugar.

Getting a medical checkup before beginning any exercise program is prudent. A screening by your physician can uncover a hidden problem like a heart defect, a tumor, or arterial blockage that needs to be addressed before you undertake any change in physical activity.

Seeing How Exercise Affects Sugar Metabolism

Some of the worst effects of a high-sugar diet are fat storage and insulin resistance (see Chapter 4). The good news is that regular exercise can reverse both of those!

Exercise improves insulin sensitivity, and it also improves your cholesterol profile. Improved function of the insulin receptors means that your body produces less insulin and stores less fat. Along with reduced carbohydrate intake, regular exercise is the most important treatment for type 2 diabetes.

Strength training is an important part of losing weight because lifting weights increases your metabolism so you burn more calories doing everything, even sitting down reading this book (stand up and keep reading!). Exercise burns up your muscles' stores of carbohydrate (called *muscle glycogen*), so when you eat carbohydrates after you work out, your body uses the carbs to refuel your muscles instead of storing them as fat. Exercise also suppresses *ghrelin* (the hunger hormone), thus decreasing your appetite and limiting cravings.

In addition to these beneficial effects on sugar metabolism, exercise reduces stress, improves brain function, reduces arthritis pain, elevates mood, improves the immune system, increases flexibility, and strengthens bones!

Sticking to an Exercise Schedule

The biggest obstacle to regular exercise is finding the time to do it. Everyone is busy, and most people overbook their schedules to the point that they don't have any time for self-care. To be healthy, this must change! Exercise doesn't take a lot of time, but you do have to be consistent to have success, which means you have to put workouts on your schedule, just like you do any other important commitment. To be successful, plan on three 30-minute blocks of exercise each week. And don't complain — I'm pretty sure you watch more than 90 minutes of TV in a week!

Setting realistic goals is an important component of success. If you tell your-self you're going to work out every day (and you don't have to, by the way), you'll either stress yourself out trying to commit that much time or feel like a failure and quit as soon as you miss a few days. Set a realistic goal of two or three half-hour blocks each week and put them on your calendar.

Your 30 minutes of exercise don't have to happen all at once. Studies show that three 10-minute bouts of exercise yield the same health improvements as one 30-minute session. The metabolic effects of just 10 minutes of exercise last at least an hour!

Reaping the Benefits of Being Consistent

Consistency is one of the most important parts of making an exercise program work for you. We live in a cause-and-effect universe, so you can't expect any improvements if you don't put in the time and effort to get them.

Exercise programming is based on the concept of *progressive overload* — taxing the body just a little bit more than it considers normal so that it's forced to adapt to the new demands that are imposed on it. That's how your body gradually gets stronger, healthier, and in better physical condition. Here are some benefits you can expect to gain from your continued progress:

- Activities of daily life improve with higher levels of fitness.
- Balance, quick reactions, and *proprioception* (body awareness) are strong deterrents to injury.
- Bone density improvements are markedly better with heavier weights and athletic moves like jumping.
- Fit people burn more fat when they exercise than unfit people.
- High levels of fitness improve your immune system.
- Higher levels of fitness open the door to more exercise options, thus avoiding boredom and burnout.
- It feels really good to be able to run as fast as your kids or to beat your husband in a push-up contest!
- Muscle content has more anti-aging impact than stress or genetics.
- You burn more calories with a higher-intensity exercise session.
- You experience more health benefits with higher levels of fitness.

Comparing Exercise Types

The exercise physiology field separates exercise into two major categories: *cardiovascular* exercise (also known as *cardio* or *aerobic* exercise) and *strength training* (also called *resistance training* or *weight training*).

Staying motivated

If you're not in great shape when you start off, staying on track with your exercise program can be a challenge. If you're a beginner, exercise isn't yet a lifestyle habit for you, so it's still something you have to plan for and put on your schedule. Your workouts may feel underwhelming or you may feel embarrassed or ashamed of how hard it is for you or how quickly you tire out. Stick with it! It gets better, I promise. Here are a few tips to help keep your motivation high:

✔ Get a friend to join the exercise program with you. Having a buddy to help you stay on track never hurts.

✔ Chart your achievements so you can see a visual representation of your progress.

✔ Share your successes on your social media accounts (Facebook, Twitter, or even set up a blog) or on the discussion boards at www.BeatingSugarAddiction.com.

✔ Read other people's success stories on blogs or support group websites (see Chapter 11). If they can do it, so can you!

Something else that may help motivate you: High-intensity workouts burn more calories than low-intensity workouts, and therefore take less time. As you get in better shape, you'll be able to work harder, so you can look forward to shorter workouts!

Fit individuals burn a greater percentage of fat for energy — 70 percent at rest versus less than 50 percent for those who are unfit. Fit people also mobilize their fat stores sooner compared to unfit people, who may take 20 to 30 minutes to tap into their fat stores. The more consistent you are with your workout plan, the better shape you get in, and the more effective your workouts get!

Cardiovascular exercise

Cardio (aerobic) exercise involves repetitive body movements that can be sustained for long periods (for many minutes or, in some cases like a marathon or the Tour de France, even hours). Cardiovascular exercise uses your body's *aerobic system* of energy, which means that it uses oxygen, stored carbohydrate, and stored fat for fuel. Examples of cardio exercise are walking, jogging, cycling, jumping rope, swimming laps, and using the stair climbers or elliptical gizmos at the gym.

Cardio exercise improves the condition of your *cardiorespiratory system* (heart, lungs, and circulatory system), burns calories, and improves glucose metabolism and insulin sensitivity.

Strength training exercise

Strength training uses an external resistance against your muscles' contractions during certain types of movements. The resistance can come from weights, exercise tubing, body weight, or any number of fun, exotic things like sandbags, medicine balls, and kettlebells. The key factor of strength training is that the resistance must be great enough to make the muscles tire after a relatively small number of contractions (typically 8 to 12 repetitions).

Strength training yields the same health benefits as cardiovascular exercise, and many additional benefits. Both burn similar numbers of calories (300 to 500 calories per typical session), but strength training is superior for a number of reasons:

✔ Strength training delivers all the health benefits of cardiovascular exercise, plus the additional benefits of increased strength, improved bone density, better flexibility, increased metabolic boost, and postural and cosmetic improvements (buff is beautiful!).

✔ Strength training results in higher *post-exercise oxygen consumption* rates (and longer durations) than cardio, meaning you burn more calories after your workout.

✔ Strength training develops your muscles, which elevates your metabolism, so you burn more calories doing everything all day.

Combining cardio and strength training

If you're pressed for time and have to pick either strength training or cardiovascular exercise, you should select strength training because you get so much more bang for your time and effort. If you have time to do both, do your workout in this order:

1. **Warm up.**

   (See *Tips for a Proper Exercise Warm-up* on www.BeatingSugar Addiction.com.)

2. **Do your strength training workout.**

3. **Do your cardio exercise.**

4. **Cool down and stretch.**

   If you need some stretching guidance, see the instructional videos at www.dummies.com/how-to/health-fitness/fitness/injury-prevention/stretching.html.

5. **Eat a protein and carbohydrate combination.**

The American College of Sports Medicine recommends that every week you should aim to burn 1,500 to 2,000 calories from exercise. That's about three hard 30-minute workouts each week. If you're not yet in good enough condition to exercise at a higher intensity, start walking every day and try to work up to being able to walk for an hour straight — that's about 300 calories. As your fitness improves, your *intensity* (how hard you exert yourself) should increase, and your exercise time can decrease.

Creating a Cardiovascular Exercise Program

Cardiovascular exercise is the simplest kind of exercise. If you walk, jog, dance, or hike, you don't need any special equipment, and you can exercise pretty much anywhere and at any time. Cardio exercise generally requires no practice or special skills, and it provides an easy way to work up a good sweat, burn some extra calories, loosen your stiff muscles, and clear your head.

Don't fall into the trap of spending a majority of your exercise time doing only cardio work. Cardio burns calories, improves your insulin sensitivity, and gets your circulatory system in better shape — all good things. But a high-intensity strength circuit (which I lay out in the section "Developing a Strength Training Workout" later in the chapter) does all that, plus it raises your metabolism, increases your strength and bone density, improves your posture, tones your muscles, burns fat, and improves your core stability and balance. Put most of your time and effort into your weight training workouts, and do cardio as an extra.

Choosing your cardio activity

As an exercise and nutrition professional, I'm often asked, "Which cardio exercise (or which cardio machine) is the best?" The answer is, "They're pretty much all the same."

The purpose of cardiovascular exercise is to elevate your heart rate and respiration for a particular length of time. Cardio doesn't tax your muscles enough to stimulate much muscular development, so asking which cardio gizmo works your legs more (or hips, or butt, or whatever body part you're trying to target) is moot. Your *level of exertion* — how high your heart rate gets and how hard you breathe — determines how many calories you burn. Whether you're jogging, cycling, using the elliptical machine, jumping rope, or swimming, the benefits are determined by how hard you exercise, not by the kind of cardio you pick.

Squeezing in extra activity

Sitting for long periods of time *(sedentary behavior)* has been shown to be a health risk all by itself, independent of exercise habits. Meeting the guidelines for physical activity doesn't negate the health risks that come from sitting all day. Time spent watching TV or working on a computer adds up and increases health risks over time. Get up and move as often as you can!

Here are some ways you can break up the monotony of sitting and increase your daily activity level without blocking out any more time:

✔ If you have a desk job, stand up and do a few stretches every 30 or 60 minutes.

✔ March in place while you watch TV or brush your teeth.

✔ Stand up (and pace if you feel like it) while you're on the phone or reading. Some companies encourage standing during meetings instead of sitting.

✔ Take the stairs instead of the elevator or escalator.

✔ When you get out of the car, walk one lap around the parking lot before you go inside (unless you're going into the gym).

The best cardio to choose is one you enjoy — or at least one you don't hate. You have hundreds of ways to exercise, so pick something you don't dread. Mix it up so you don't get bored.

Determining duration and frequency

As of the time of this writing, here are the current guidelines for cardiovascular exercise from the American College of Sports Medicine, the leading organization for publishing exercise research and establishing exercise guidelines:

✔ Adults should get at least 150 minutes of moderate-intensity exercise per week.

✔ You can meet exercise recommendations through 30 to 60 minutes of moderate-intensity exercise five days per week or 20 to 60 minutes of vigorous-intensity exercise three days per week.

✔ One continuous session and multiple shorter sessions (of at least 10 minutes) are both acceptable ways to accumulate the desired amount of daily exercise.

✔ Gradual progression of exercise time, frequency, and intensity is recommended for continued motivation and the least risk of injury.

Any exercise is better than none! If you're unable to meet these minimums, you can still benefit from some activity. Do *something!*

Finding the right difficulty level

The difficulty or intensity of cardiovascular exercise is determined by how high your heart rate gets. When gauging the intensity of your cardio exercise, you can either assess how hard you feel like you're working (self-perception) or get more precise and measure your actual pulse rate.

If you'd like to keep things simple, use a scale of 1 to 10 during your cardio exercise to describe how hard you feel like you're working:

>   1 = Am I lying in a hammock or am I exercising?

>   3 = I'm doing something but it's very, very easy.

>   5 = This isn't too hard; I could do this for at least an hour. (Activities may include walking, hiking, or yardwork, for example.)

>   7 = I'm working pretty hard. I'll tire out relatively soon.

>   10 = I'm exerting the absolute maximum effort I can before I pass out or my heart explodes.

Here's how to determine your pulse rate: Using your index and middle fingers, find your pulse, either on your neck next to your windpipe or on your wrist straight down from your index finger. Count the beats for 10 seconds, and then multiply that number by 6 to get your *beats per minute* (bpm).

While you're at rest, your normal heart rate should range from the low 50s to about 85 bpm. In general, the better condition you're in, the lower your resting heart rate is because your heart and vascular system are more efficient.

You can make it your goal to keep your heart rate elevated to a specific target number, known as your *target heart rate,* and keep it there for a predetermined amount of time. While doing your cardiovascular exercise, stop and check your pulse rate periodically to determine whether you're working at your target heart rate. If your heart rate is below your target range, pick up the pace. If it's too high, slow down so you can stay in your target range.

To determine your target heart rate, you must first calculate your predicted maximum heart rate, which is 208 minus 70 percent of your age. That's the estimated maximum speed your heart can beat. If you're 46 years old, your predicted maximum heart rate is 176 beats per minute: 70 percent of 46 is 32; 208 – 32 = 176. Unless you're running away from a grizzly bear, you don't need to exercise at your absolute maximum effort, so you find your target heart rate by taking a percentage of your predicted maximum:

>   ✔ 50 to 60 percent if you're very out of shape or on heart medication

✔ 70 to 85 percent for general fitness conditioning ("getting in shape")

✔ 90 to 100 percent for high-intensity intervals or sport-specific athletic training

Using the example of a 46-year-old, the target heart rate ranges (in beats per minute) would be:

✔ 88 to 106 bpm (50 to 60 percent of 176) for those who are very out of shape or on heart medication

✔ 123 to 150 bpm (70 to 85 percent of 176) for general fitness conditioning

✔ 158 to 176 bpm (90 to 100 percent of 176) for high-intensity intervals or sport-specific athletic training

 Certain medical conditions or prescription medications can artificially suppress your heart rate. If you have any medical conditions or take medication that affects your heart rate (medications for blood pressure, most commonly), you should get some professional help to set up a safe and appropriate exercise program (see the sidebar "Finding a fitness trainer" later in this chapter).

Structuring your cardio exercise

You can structure your cardio exercise in two ways: *steady-state exercise* or *interval training*.

✔ **Steady-state cardiovascular exercise** means that you exercise at a certain pace (or a certain target heart rate), and you stay there for a predetermined length of time. If you're new to exercise, I recommend you start with steady-state cardio because it's easier. You don't want to over-stress your joints and muscles with high-intensity exercise that you're not yet conditioned for.

Your goal should be a cardio workout that lasts somewhere between 10 minutes and 60 minutes, depending on your intensity and your fitness levels. Work at a level of difficulty between 5 (very manageable) and 8 (pretty hard) or use the target heart rate system if you prefer (see the preceding section for an explanation of these difficulty levels and target heart rate).

✔ **Interval training** is a more difficult version of cardiovascular exercise. You take a standard steady-state workout and sprinkle in high-intensity intervals of near-maximum effort. With interval training, you get more work done in less time, you burn more calories, you get better fitness benefits, and you get a longer *afterburn*, meaning that your metabolism stays elevated for a longer time after your workout.

Here's an example of a 20-minute cardiovascular workout using interval training:

1. Three minutes at level 3 (very easy) as a warm-up

2. Twenty to sixty seconds of near-maximum work (level 9 to 10)

3. Three minutes at level 5 for recovery

4. Repeat Steps 2 and 3 three more times (four total intervals)

5. Three minutes at level 3 for a cool-down

I usually recommend that most people aim to incorporate interval training as soon as they're physically and medically able because it yields more health and fitness benefits, requires shorter workouts, and keeps you from getting bored. However, steady-state workouts are preferable to some people. Maybe you enjoy the peace and meditative state that can come from a steady-state jog or cycling workout. Perhaps you enjoy doing cardio with a friend or a running group and use the time as much for socializing as you do for exercise. Whatever your reason to pick one over the other, the most important things are that you do it, you enjoy it, and you stay consistent with your workouts!

Watching out for trouble

One of the downsides to any repetitive activity (like cardio) is that it leaves you vulnerable to overuse injuries like tendinitis, bursitis, and stress fractures. Here are some tips to help you stay injury-free:

- **Vary your activity frequently.** Performing a variety of activities utilizes the muscles differently and helps limit overuse of any one system. Take a break from the treadmill and use the bike instead. Get outside and play tennis or shoot some basketball. If you're a jogger, mix up your routes so you don't run the same terrain every day. Variety keeps both your body and your brain fresh!

- **Recognize signs of overuse.** Stay on the lookout for consistently irritated muscles, reduced physical performance, sluggishness, achy joints, or frequent illness. If you experience any of these symptoms, listen to your body and take a few days off to see whether that helps rejuvenate you.

- **Stretch regularly throughout the day.** Having certain muscles that are too tight is asking for injury. Get an evaluation from a good physical therapist or qualified exercise professional to find out what you need to stretch and how to do it.

- **Don't overdo it.** The key to long-term success is to be consistent, with a gradual progression of overload and physical challenges. Use a sensible progression of increasing time or intensity — don't try to get in shape in a week!

Developing a Strength Training Workout

Strength training — working out with weights or other resistance equipment like exercise tubing, medicine balls, sandbags, or suspension straps — increases strength, improves flexibility, raises metabolism, improves immunity, increases bone density, improves balance and day-to-day function, increases insulin response, and boosts energy. Plus it's fun!

Choosing the right exercises

A comprehensive strength training program needs to incorporate the six basic types of body movements that utilize all the major muscle groups. Although it's tempting to seek out exercises that target your so-called problem areas, exercising particular muscles doesn't burn fat away from that specific area; that's a myth called *spot reduction.* When your body pulls out fat for fuel, it takes it from wherever it pleases, and unfortunately, you have no control over where that is. Being able to decide where the fat comes off would be great, but your body doesn't work that way. Exercise and proper nutrition make you lose fat, but you can't decide where.

The following list shows the six major types of exercises that should make up the foundation of your strength training workouts. I cover proper form and exercise technique later in this chapter. The specific variations and the level of difficulty of these exercises that you choose depend on your abilities and your goals. This is where some professional guidance would be beneficial; check out the sidebar "Finding a fitness trainer" later in the chapter.

- **Triple-extension movements** are multi-joint leg exercises like squats, lunges, step-ups, and leg presses. They work all the muscles of the thighs and hips.

- **Pushing movements** work the chest, shoulders, and arms. Examples are push-ups, bench presses, and chest flies.

- **Pulling movements** work the back, shoulders, neck, and arms. Examples are rows, chin-ups, pull-downs, and reverse flies. Pulling exercises are essential for correct posture.

- **Core exercises** focus on the midsection — waist, trunk, and pelvis. A strong core is essential for spinal stability and the prevention of back injuries. Examples of core exercises are crunches, sit-ups, planks, twists, and back extensions.

- **Overhead movements,** like the overhead press and the lateral raise, work the shoulders and arms.

> ✔ **Posterior chain movements** target the group of muscles behind you — the hamstrings, glutes, and spinal erectors (the lower back muscles). Exercises that work the posterior chain are dead lifts, bridges, and hip extensions.

For more detailed information about what muscles do and which exercises work which muscles, see the *Muscles Overview* article posted on www. BeatingSugarAddiction.com.

Figuring sets and reps for optimal results

Following are a couple of definitions so that when exercise stuff comes up in conversation with your friends, you can sound like you know what you're talking about.

When you execute an exercise move one time, that's called a *repetition,* or *rep* for short. When you do a bunch of repetitions in a row, that group of reps is called a *set.* Suppose you're doing the Romanian dead lift for the posterior chain — you do it 12 times before you tire out, you rest a minute, and then you do it another 12 times. The way you describe what you did is to say you did *two sets of 12 reps.* Congratulations — now you sound like a workout veteran!

If you're into fitness magazines or blogs, you'll find a gazillion variations of sets and reps options out there. To simplify things, here are some very basic guidelines for beginners: Start with one set of each of the six basic exercise movements in the preceding section, and pick a weight or a level of difficulty that allows you to perform 15 to 20 repetitions. As your strength and abilities improve, gradually increase both the number of sets and the difficulty of the exercise, and work your way up to three or four sets of 8 to 10 repetitions.

Balancing strength training and recovery time

When you tax your muscles with strength training, they need some time to recover and rebuild. The harder you work your muscles, the more recovery time they need. Give yourself at least 48 hours of recovery between workouts with weights — or more if you're still sore.

Your body makes muscle and bone improvements while you're resting, not while you work out. If you don't give yourself adequate recovery time, you won't get the desired *physiological adaptations,* and you can start to experience signs of overtraining — consistent soreness and fatigue, poor muscular performance, and overuse injuries like tendinitis. Being motivated is great, but don't overdo it! For most folks, three 30-minute resistance training workouts each week should be plenty.

Performing Basic Strength Training Exercises Correctly

Proper form is important for getting the most out of your strength workouts, and it's also essential for staying free of injuries. In addition to reading through the descriptions and instructions presented in this section, I strongly suggest that you get at least a few lessons from a qualified exercise professional, both to teach you correct execution of the exercises and to determine which variations and levels of difficulty are appropriate for you. See the sidebar "Finding a fitness trainer" later in this chapter for some tips on seeking out professional exercise instruction.

Exercises for the thighs, glutes, and hips

The thighs and hips are some of the largest and strongest muscles in your body. They're responsible for moving you around all day, and they're the driving force when you stand, sit, walk, run, jump, squat down, and go up and down stairs. Keeping your legs strong is especially important for the aging population to keep good mobility and to prevent falls.

Squat

The *squat* (see Figure 12-1) is one of the fundamental functional exercise moves. More than 200 muscles are active when you do a squat, and it has many practical carry-overs to daily life. You need to master the squat before tackling the more advanced, single-leg moves like lunges or step-ups.

Start with your feet shoulder-width apart and angled out slightly, with your heels planted firmly on the floor. Keeping your back muscles tight and the shape of your spine the same, start to lean your pelvis and upper body forward as you begin to bend your knees, like you're starting to sit down into a chair. If you look at yourself from the side, your shoulder should be over your ankle. Continue bending your knees and sinking your hips down until (ideally) your thighs are parallel to the ground. Press your heels into the floor and drive yourself back up to the standing position.

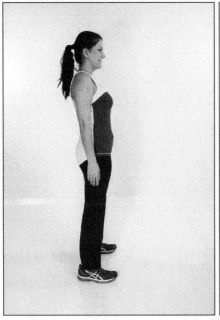
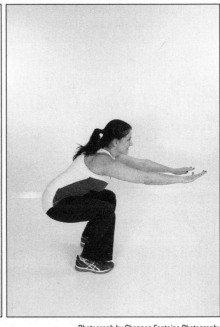

Figure 12-1:
Squat.

Photograph by Shannon Fontaine Photography

 If a full squat (thighs parallel to the floor) is too hard or if you're not flexible enough to get down all the way, stick with a shorter squat — try just half-way down — until your strength and flexibility improve. On the other hand, if squatting with just your body weight gets too easy, hold some dumbbells while you do it or add a five-second hold at the bottom of each rep. Or both!

 Feel free to practice this move with some balance assistance until you feel confident; try squatting with your butt against a wall until you feel like you can keep your balance without help. Alternatively, you can try holding onto a chair or a broomstick with your arms while you squat.

Lunge

A *lunge* (see Figure 12-2) is a more difficult version of the squat because most of your weight is on one leg. Begin standing with your feet underneath your hip sockets. Shift your weight onto one leg and slide the other foot approximately 2 feet behind you. Keeping your weight on the heel of your front foot, begin to squat, bending both knees and leaning your upper body forward (just like a squat) so that your shoulder stays over your front ankle. When your back knee touches the floor, press your front heel into the floor and pull yourself forward into the standing position. Be sure to keep your front knee over your ankle — don't let your thigh roll inward. Do some reps on one leg and then switch sides. Don't be surprised if one side is significantly harder than the other.

Figure 12-2:
Lunge.

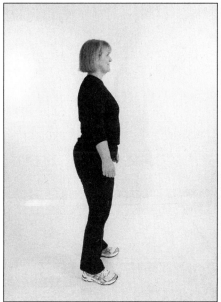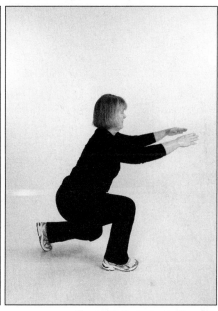

Photograph by Shannon Fontaine Photography

The lunge has many variations, like forward lunges, walking lunges, and side lunges. Master this version (stepping back into the lunge position) before you try any others.

Lying hip adduction

The *lying hip adduction* (see Figure 12-3) is an exercise for the inner thigh muscles. Lie on your side, bend your top knee, and plant your top foot flat on the floor in front of your bottom knee. Flex your inner thigh muscles on your bottom leg to lift your bottom leg off the ground. Hold for one second and then lower. Repeat reps on one side and then flip over and do the other leg.

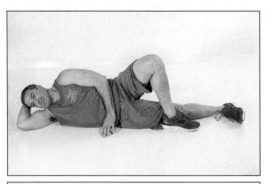

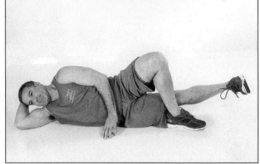

Figure 12-3:
Lying hip
adduction.

Photograph by Shannon Fontaine Photography

Lying hip abduction

The *lying hip abduction* (see Figure 12-4) is the opposite move of the lying hip adduction. Lie on your side with your bottom knee bent and your top leg straight and parallel to your spine (it will feel like it's behind you). Flex your foot (pull your toes up toward your shin) and turn your top thigh one click outward so that your kneecap and foot point a little bit upward instead of straight ahead. Lift your top leg approximately 45 degrees, hold for one second, and slowly lower. Do your reps on one hip and then flip over and do the other side. Like the lunge, you'll probably find that one hip is weaker than the other. If that's the case, do one set on the weak side, one set on the stronger side, and a second set on the weaker side to bring it up to snuff.

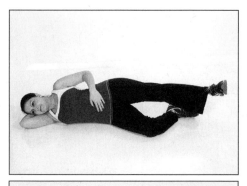

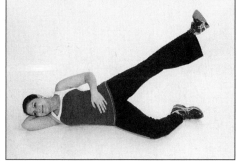

Figure 12-4:
Lying hip
abduction.

Photograph by Shannon Fontaine Photography

Exercises for the posterior chain

Strengthening your hamstrings, glutes, and lower back muscles is important for avoiding injury and chronic back pain. Mastering these exercises is also good training for keeping proper spine mechanics when you're lifting things or bending over to pick up stuff.

Bridge

To perform the *bridge* (see Figure 12-5), lie on your back with your knees bent, your heels planted on the floor, and your feet flexed up off the ground. Brace your trunk with your core muscles so you can keep your spine from changing shape while you do the move. Press your heels down into the floor to drive your hips up toward the ceiling. Squeeze your glutes (butt muscles) and don't overarch your lower back — the shape of your spine shouldn't change while you bridge. Hold the top of the bridge for one second and then slowly lower.

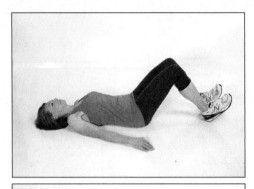

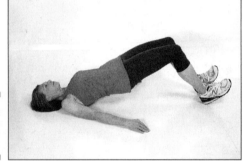

Figure 12-5:
Hamstring
bridge.

Photograph by Shannon Fontaine Photography

More advanced variations of the bridge include putting your feet on an exercise ball or doing the bridge with one leg instead of two. Or, if you're really getting strong, both!

Romanian dead lift

One of my favorite exercises for the posterior chain is the *Romanian dead lift* (see Figure 12-6). It's a very functional, practical exercise for strengthening the back and ingraining proper lifting mechanics.

Holding a pair of dumbbells, start in a standing position with your knees unlocked and your feet about 6 inches apart. Tighten your back muscles to put a little arch in your back, and lean forward from your hips, keeping your back nice and tight. Don't allow your spine to round or your shoulders to hump over. When you can no longer tilt your pelvis any farther (your hamstrings will reach their end range of motion), stop and pull yourself back up to the standing position.

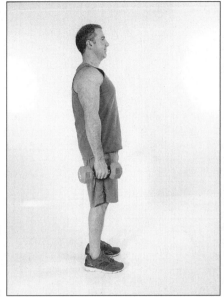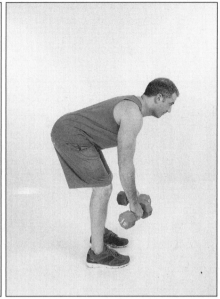

Figure 12-6:
Romanian
dead lift.

Photograph by Shannon Fontaine Photography

Exercises for the shoulders and arms

Keeping your arms and shoulders in good shape helps make you stronger for your daily activities. Doing so also makes you look great in T-shirts and sleeveless dresses!

Overhead press

The basic exercise for your shoulders is the *overhead press* (see Figure 12-7). Start in a standing position with your knees unlocked, your elbows bent so your forearms are perpendicular to the floor, and your upper arms at your sides. Drive your arms up to the vertical position (touchdown!) so your elbows are in line with your ears. Don't overarch your back; leave your hips over your heels. Slowly lower your elbows back down to your sides.

Push-ups

Push-ups (see Figure 12-8) are a good way to strengthen your chest, arms, and shoulders. Start on your knees with your hands slightly wider than shoulder-width apart. Keep your hips down so there's a straight line between your knees and your head. Bend your elbows and pull your shoulder blades together to lower your body until your chest touches the floor. Your arms should be approximately 45 degrees out from your ribs. Flex your chest and arm muscles to press yourself back to the straight-arm position.

Biceps curl

The *biceps* are the muscles on the front of the upper arm that bend your elbow. To perform the *biceps curl* (see Figure 12-9), start in a standing position holding dumbbells with your palms facing forward. Bend both elbows, pulling your palms toward your shoulders. Try not to let your elbows swing forward at the top; keep them at your ribs. Squeeze your biceps one second at the top and then slowly straighten your arms back to the starting position. Straighten your arms all the way at the bottom.

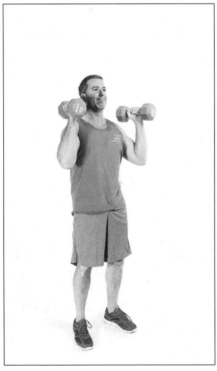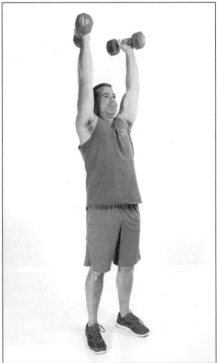

Figure 12-7:
Overhead
press.

Photograph by Shannon Fontaine Photography

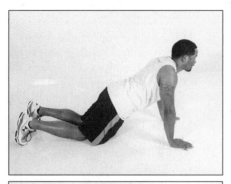

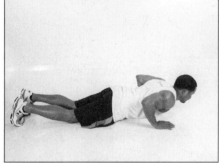

Figure 12-8:
Push-up.

Photograph by Shannon Fontaine Photography

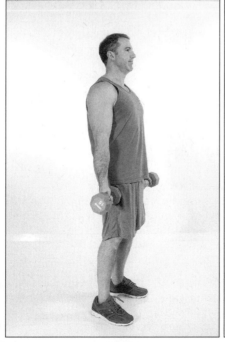

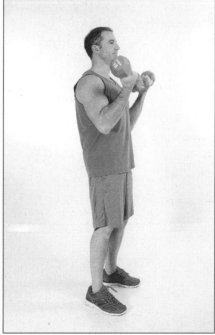

Figure 12-9:
Biceps curl.

Photograph by Shannon Fontaine Photography

Lying triceps extension

To work the backs of your arms, grab some dumbbells and start the *lying triceps extension* (see Figure 12-10) on your back, with your knees bent and your arms straight up toward the ceiling. Keeping your elbows fixed on an imaginary board or shelf, bend both elbows, lowering your hands to your ears. Be careful not to hit yourself in the head with the weights! Flex your triceps to straighten your arms back to the starting position.

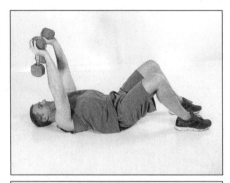

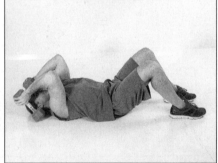

Figure 12-10:
Lying triceps extension.

Photograph by Shannon Fontaine Photography

Pulling exercises for the back

Keeping the upper back muscles strong is important for good posture and for preventing chronic neck and shoulder pain. Most people who sit a lot need extra work in this area. In your workouts, be sure to do at least as much pulling as you do pushing, if not more.

Standing tubing row

The *standing tubing row* (see Figure 12-11) is a great way to strengthen your upper back and improve your posture. Grab your exercise tubing and insert the anchor into the hinge side of the door (if you've never used exercise tubing before, the website www.BeatingSugarAddiction.com has a quick how-to video). Stand facing the anchor and split your feet so you're braced with one foot ahead of the other. Begin with both arms straight ahead, palms facing each other. Squeeze your shoulder blades together and pull your elbows back, keeping your forearms parallel to the floor. The end position is your shoulder blades squeezed in toward your spine and down away from your ears. Hold the squeeze for one second and then reverse the move back to the starting position.

Figure 12-11:
Standing
tubing row.

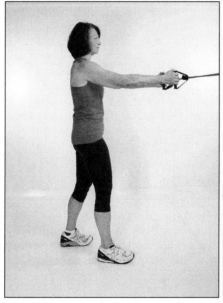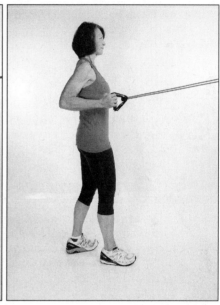

Photograph by Shannon Fontaine Photography

Single-arm row

Another common variation of the row is the *single-arm row* (see Figure 12-12). Start standing with a dumbbell in one hand. Step forward with the opposite leg and lean forward with a straight spine (no rounding), resting the non-dumbbell hand on your forward thigh. Perform the rowing movement on the dumbbell side just like you perform the standing row — pull your shoulder blade back toward your spine and pull your arm back, keeping your forearm perpendicular to the ground. Try not to twist your upper body as you pull. Hold the retracted position for one second and then return to the starting position.

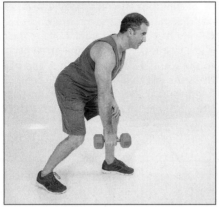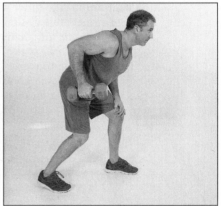

Photograph by Shannon Fontaine Photography

Figure 12-12:
Single-arm
row.

If you find it too difficult to keep your back correct when doing the leaning-over version, try putting your knee and hand (the nonworking side) on a bench, chair, or exercise ball instead.

Core exercises for the abs and waist

Remember that exercising your abdominal muscles doesn't burn fat away from that area! Smart eating and consistent exercise create the physiological environment and caloric deficit needed to lose body fat. You can't pick where your fat comes off, and you can't out-exercise a bad diet!

U crunch

The *U crunch* (see Figure 12-13) is a core exercise that strengthens the abdominals and stretches the lower back. Start by lying on your back with your feet up, your knees bent, and your arms up toward the ceiling. Flex your abdominal muscles to curl your spine forward so that your chest and ribs pull down toward your navel and your pelvis rolls back toward your ribs. Aim for half the movement to come from your upper body and half from the pelvis roll. Hold the contracted position for one second and then unroll back to the starting position. Be careful not to overarch your lower back in the starting position.

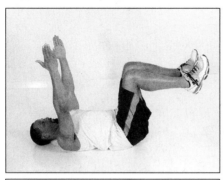

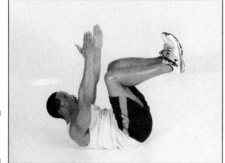

Figure 12-13:
U crunch.

Photograph by Shannon Fontaine Photography

Seated twist

The *seated twist* (see Figure 12-14) strengthens the waist and targets the twisting muscles — primarily your *obliques* and *spinal erectors.* Start seated on the floor with your knees bent. Crunch your stomach muscles (pulling your ribs down and rolling your pelvis back) so your lower back is rounded. Rock back onto your tailbone, maintaining a rounded lower back. Slowly twist your upper body approximately 45 degrees from side to side until you can't hold the position anymore. If your back hurts before your abs, you've lost your rounded shape. If using just body weight is too easy, hold a medicine ball or dumbbell while you twist.

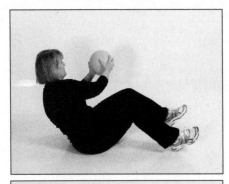

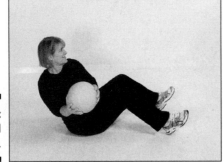

Figure 12-14:
Seated
twist.

Photograph by Shannon Fontaine Photography

Plank

The *plank* (see Figure 12-15) is one of the mainstays of core stabilization exercises. The goal is to be able to stiffen your spine like a board or a plank and hold it in the same shape in a variety of positions.

To begin the basic plank, start on all fours and then walk your hands forward until the line between your knees and your head is straight (like a plank). Flex your abdominal muscles and roll your pelvis under so your lower back is rounded. Hold your spine in that shape and go down onto your elbows where your hands were. Just hold still and breathe. Feel your abs?

If you can hold this position for 15 seconds and it's not difficult, lift up onto your toes instead of your knees (see Figure 12-16). Just like in the seated twist, if your back hurts instead of your abs, you've lost your rounded lower back.

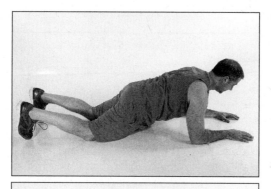

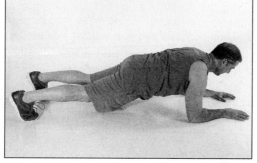

Figure 12-15: Plank on knees and toes.

Photograph by Shannon Fontaine Photography

A common variation of this exercise is the *side plank* (see Figure 12-16). Start lying on your side with your feet stacked on top of each other and your bottom forearm on the floor. Lift your hips to form a straight line from feet to head.

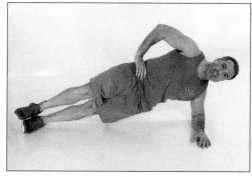

Figure 12-16: Side plank.

Photograph by Shannon Fontaine Photography

Finding a fitness trainer

Because everyone's body is different and everyone learns differently, I recommend that you hire a qualified exercise instructor to help you put together a safe and effective exercise program to reach your goals.

You can find multitudes of gyms and private exercise studios, all of which have fitness trainers available. Sadly, the fact that someone holds a fitness certification doesn't mean that he or she is a well-educated, qualified teacher. Instead of hiring just anyone, do some homework first to make sure that you find the best teacher available in your area.

If you know some local health and wellness providers (massage therapists, physicians, chiropractors, or physical therapists), ask whom they'd recommend for fitness instruction.

Barring that, call some personal trainers and ask, "If I can't work with you (or someone in your company), whom do you suggest I hire?" If you get the same name more than once, chances are you have a winner.

To make a blanket statement, if you need help with basic fitness programming (losing weight and getting in shape), your trainer should put you on a system relatively similar to what I've outlined in this chapter. If you're new to exercise and your personal trainer starts you off with a bodybuilding-style split routine on your first week (chest and arms on one day, legs on another day, and so on), find a different trainer who's more versed in functional fitness and modern exercise programming.

Putting It All Together: Sample Workouts

You can do countless variations of workouts, so you'll never be bored. This section includes two examples to get you started: an easy workout and a difficult one.

Example workout 1 (easy)

Warm-up: Five to ten minutes of light activity of your choice — treadmill, elliptical, seated rowing machine, stationary bike, marching in place, and so on.

Strength training portion: One set of 15 to 20 repetitions of each of these six exercises, with approximately a minute rest in between sets:

1. Squats
2. Push-ups
3. Standing rows with tubing

4. Bridges

5. Overhead presses with dumbbells

6. Planks or U crunches

Cardiovascular portion: Twenty to thirty minutes of the cardio exercise of your choice at low to medium intensity: 60 to 75 percent of (208 – 70 percent of your age).

Five-minute cool-down: Low-intensity version of the cardio you were doing, or just walking.

Flexibility: Stretch your three or four tightest areas for 30 seconds, two times each. Don't forget to breathe!

Example workout 2 (difficult)

Warm-up: Five to ten minutes of light activity of your choice — treadmill, elliptical, seated rowing machine, stationary bike, marching in place, and so on.

Strength training portion: Perform one set of 8 to 10 repetitions of each of these six exercises, with very little rest between exercises. When you've gone through all six, rest for about two minutes and then repeat the list. After two rounds, see whether you have a third round in you!

1. Lunges (8 to 10 on each leg)

2. Push-ups

3. Single-arm rows with dumbbell (8 to 10 each side)

4. Romanian dead lifts

5. Dumbbell curls into overhead presses

6. Seated twists with a medicine ball or dumbbell

Cardiovascular portion: Fifteen minutes of the cardio exercise of your choice at medium to high intensity: 75 to 90 percent of (208 – 70 percent of your age).

Five-minute cool-down: Low-intensity version of the cardio you were doing, or just walking.

Flexibility: Stretch your three or four tightest areas for 30 seconds, two times each. Don't forget to breathe!

Part IV
Sugar-Busting Recipes

Five Easy Substitutions for Healthier Eating

✔ **Drink mineral water instead of soda.** Mineral water flavored with citrus will give you the fizz and the flavor that you love without the sugar and chemicals that come with soda. Staying hydrated can help stave off sugar cravings, too!

✔ **Use stevia instead of sugar or artificial sweeteners.** Stevia is a plant whose powder is used as a natural, no-calorie sweetener. Stevia has a negligible effect on your blood sugar, and it doesn't have the possible health hazards associated with chemical sweeteners.

✔ **Snack on raw veggies instead of junk food.** Keeping fresh raw veggies ready to snack on will make it easy for you to make the smart choice when you need to nibble. Crunching on low-calorie, high-nutrient vegetables will satisfy your hunger and add valuable nutrition to your daily diet.

✔ **Choose organic whole grains like oats, rice, and spelt instead of white flour.** Whole grains are chock-full of B vitamins and minerals. The fiber from whole grains helps you feel full and helps keep your blood sugar and insulin levels from spiking too fast. White flour digests quickly and causes a more rapid rise in blood sugar, followed by a sugar crash that leads to hunger and cravings.

✔ **Buy pasture-raised eggs and meat instead of feedlot products.** Animals raised in commercial feedlots are kept in overcrowded conditions and are fed industrial feed containing chemicals, hormones, and antibiotics. Meat, dairy, and eggs from these animals contain these contaminants. Pasture-raised animals are treated more humanely and have access to a healthy, natural diet, yielding healthier food.

Starting your day with a good breakfast elevates your metabolism and helps keep you from overeating later in the day. Find free recommendations for best breakfast practices at www.dummies.com/extras/beatingsugaraddiction.

In this part . . .

- ✔ Start the day off right by going beyond the cereal box with protein-packed, low-sugar breakfasts.

- ✔ Prevent midday slumps by making smart lunch choices loaded with veggies and healthy protein.

- ✔ Fortify your family with speedy dinner recipes ranging from creative seafood options to more traditional meat and vegetarian dishes.

- ✔ Satisfy cravings with healthy snacks that fill you up without sabotaging your low-sugar goals.

- ✔ Redefine desserts to get the satisfaction you want with less sugar and more flavor.

Chapter 13

Energy-Boosting Breakfasts

In This Chapter

▶ Understanding why breakfast is so important

▶ Keeping sugar in your breakfast to a minimum

An old saying advises, "Eat breakfast like a king, lunch like a prince, and dinner like a pauper," but many Americans do the opposite. Under-eating during the day and overeating at night is exactly the wrong way to eat if you're trying to lose weight. Doing so also works against you if you're trying to keep your energy up and your mental performance sharp. When you wake up in the morning, you've gone eight or ten hours without food, your body is craving nourishment, and your brain needs glucose to function at its best. Skipping breakfast is one of the worst possible things you can do — you set yourself up for fatigue, poor mental acuity, and sugar cravings later in the day.

Appreciating the Importance of Breakfast

People who eat breakfast are far more likely to get a healthy intake of vitamins and minerals than those who don't. In one study published in the *Journal of the American College of Nutrition,* researchers found that people who ate a hearty breakfast containing more than 25 percent of their daily calories had a higher intake of essential vitamins and minerals — and lower cholesterol levels, too!

Research shows that between 35 and 40 percent of Americans skip breakfast, and many kids leave for school without it. The implications are dramatic, both physically and mentally. People who skip breakfast are more than four times as likely to be obese than people who eat something in the morning. Skipping breakfast makes you fatter!

Thinking outside the cereal box

When some people sit down for breakfast, they automatically grab a quick, all-carbohydrate food like breakfast cereal or a muffin. Don't be afraid to think outside the American breakfast food box — even the recommended high-protein breakfast can get stale if you're stuck on just eggs and sausage. A traditional Japanese breakfast consists of a small piece of fish (like salmon), some light vegetables, and a tiny portion of rice accompanied by a small bowl of miso soup. The health benefits of fish and vegetables in the morning are huge, and the omega-3 fats (see Chapter 5) in salmon are terrific for your skin, help regulate mood, and are essential for proper hormone formation. If breakfasting on fish or other leftovers is too much of a stretch for you, consider these options:

✔ A cup of organic Greek yogurt with nuts, grapes, or berries: Greek yogurt contains active probiotic cultures (beneficial bacteria — see Chapter 5) and has twice the protein and half the carbs as regular yogurt.

✔ Natural peanut or almond butter on a slice of whole-grain bread: Fold it in half and enjoy your easy, no-cook breakfast. A nut butter sandwich goes great with a glass of skim milk or some hot green tea.

✔ A low-sugar whey protein shake: It's fast, inexpensive, and versatile, and it has the protein you may be used to getting from bacon, sausage, and eggs. You can mix a scoop of whey powder in milk or diluted juice or blend a smoothie by mixing a scoop or two of whey with a handful of frozen berries or half a banana. Try powdered whey in a splash of cranberry juice, pomegranate juice, almond milk, or rice milk. Adding a teaspoon of flax oil to the shake adds essential fats and helps the smoothie stick with you a little longer. Experiment and see what you like!

Numerous studies over the years have shown that skipping breakfast affects the behavior and mental performance of children in school, too. Kids who eat breakfast have better memory and higher math and reading scores. Kids who are hungry have a higher number of behavior problems, including fighting, stealing, having difficulty with teachers, and not acknowledging rules.

Launching Your Day the Low-Sugar Way

The traditional continental breakfast is typically an all-carbohydrate affair. Plates loaded with muffins, bagels, breakfast cereals, and pastries cause a giant rush of sugar into the body, with the corresponding insulin crash several hours later.

The ideal breakfast has a high protein content. Higher-protein breakfasts translate into a more sustained level of energy throughout the morning (no carb crash). Protein fills you up longer, meaning you're less likely to have midmorning cravings. You're also less likely to overeat at lunch or to get so hungry during the day that you grab whatever is available in the break room or the vending machine. More protein at breakfast also increases metabolism; in one study, a high-protein breakfast *doubled* the metabolism of healthy young women!

Traditional protein sources for breakfast include eggs, ham, sausage, yogurt, and whey. You have plenty of other options, though — don't get stuck in a breakfast rut!

Don't eat the same thing for breakfast every day. Eating a variety of foods means that you get a wider spectrum of nutrients. Changing up the breakfast routine also makes the meal more appealing for those who may not like to eat in the morning.

Eggs: Good or bad?

Some published research has concluded that the consumption of eggs (or red meat) raises your risk of cardiovascular disease — atherosclerosis, heart attacks, strokes, and so on. After reviewing the current research available and having an understanding of how the body's inflammatory response affects the cardiovascular system, I think that the bad rap given to eggs and red meat is due to the quality and origin of the food itself.

Eating food produced from sick animals that are fed chemically enhanced, genetically modified grain raises the level of inflammation in your body. Garbage in, garbage out, as they say. Almost all research reporting that red meat and eggs are bad for your cardiovascular health has been done with food from commercial feedlot animals. The nutrition profile for healthy animal products (organic and pasture-fed) is much better, and these foods don't cause the high inflammatory response that the industrial feedlot products do.

According to the American Egg Board, 60 commercial egg producers have over 1 million hens in gigantic factory housing. Twelve of them have over 5 million! These unthinkably crowded living conditions are the reason that commercial producers use antibiotics in their chicken feed and why industrial eggs must be bathed in chemicals to sanitize them. I recommend pasture-fed, antibiotic-free eggs because pasture feeding gives eggs a higher nutrient content than conventional eggs, is better for the chickens, and doesn't perpetuate antibiotic resistance like conventional chicken feed does.

Eggs are loaded with protein and other nutrients, such as phosphatidyl choline for the brain and lutein and zeaxanthin for the eyes. If you need to lower the amount of fat in your diet, you can use egg whites instead of whole eggs, but if you do, remember that you're missing out on a lot of important nutrients in the pasture-fed yolks.

Protein Muffins

Prep time: 10 min • **Cook time:** 20–25 min • **Yield:** 8 large muffins (or 12 smaller muffins)

Ingredients	Directions
2 tablespoons canola oil	*1* Preheat the oven to 375 degrees. In a muffin pan, line 8 cups with paper muffin liners. (This recipe makes 8 large or 12 small muffins, so use the number of liners based on the size you desire.)
1½ cups unsweetened applesauce	
1 cup unbleached white flour	
1 cup whole-wheat flour	*2* In a large mixing bowl, beat together the egg, oil, and applesauce with an electric mixer on low speed.
¾ teaspoon baking soda	
2 teaspoons baking powder	*3* Add the flour, baking soda, baking powder, whey powder, walnuts, and spices. Beat well on medium speed. Stir in the raisins.
1½ scoops unsweetened whey protein powder (about 2 tablespoons)	
¼ cup chopped walnuts	*4* Spoon the batter into the prepared muffin pan. Bake for 20 to 25 minutes, or until well-browned and firm to the touch.
½ teaspoon nutmeg	
½ teaspoon cinnamon	
¾ cup raisins	*5* Cool on wire racks.

Per serving: Calories 241 (From Fat 7); Fat 7g (Saturated 0.5g); Cholesterol 1mg; Sodium 121mg; Carbohydrate 41g (Dietary Fiber 3.5g); Protein 5g.

Tip: Serve these protein muffins warm, topped with organic cream cheese.

Multigrain Pancakes

Prep time: 20 min • **Cook time:** 8 min • **Yield:** 8 servings (16–24 pancakes)

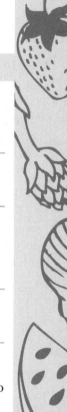

Ingredients	Directions
1¾ cups spelt flour	*1* Whisk the spelt flour, oat flour, baking powder, flaxseed meal, whey protein, and salt together in a large mixing bowl.
2 cups oat flour	
2 tablespoons baking powder	
¼ cup ground flaxseed meal	*2* In a separate bowl, stir together the soy milk, applesauce, and vanilla extract.
1½ scoops unsweetened whey protein powder (about 2 tablespoons)	
½ teaspoon salt	*3* Gradually pour the soy milk mixture into the flour mix, continually stirring them together. Stir until the ingredients are just moistened. Set aside for 15 minutes.
3½ cups low-fat vanilla soy milk	
¼ cup unsweetened applesauce	*4* Lightly butter and heat a griddle or large skillet to medium heat.
1½ tablespoons vanilla extract	
1 tablespoon butter	*5* Spoon the batter onto the hot griddle or skillet in 3- to 4-inch diameter pancakes. Sprinkle blueberries onto the wet batter, and cook until bubbles form (2 to 3 minutes). Flip the pancakes and continue cooking until golden brown on both sides, about 3 minutes more.
1½ cups blueberries, washed	
Dash of cinnamon	
	6 Serve with butter, a sprinkle of cinnamon, and the low-sugar topping of your choice.

Per serving: Calories 254 (From Fat 4.5); Fat 2.5g (Saturated 0.5g); Cholesterol 3.0mg; Sodium 102mg; Carbohydrate 24g (Dietary Fiber 3.5g); Protein 5.0g.

Tip: Good low-sugar substitutes for pancake syrup include mango spread or unsweetened applesauce mixed with a drizzle of honey.

Muesli

Prep time: 12 min • **Yield:** 12 servings (1 cup each)

Ingredients	*Directions*
4½ **cups rolled oats**	**1** Combine all ingredients except the almond milk in a large mixing bowl. Mix well and transfer to an airtight container for storage.
½ **cup toasted wheat germ**	
½ **cup wheat bran**	
½ **cup oat bran**	**2** To prepare the muesli hot, add the almond milk and microwave for 30 to 45 seconds; stir well and enjoy. To prepare the muesli cold, just add the milk and mix it up with a spoon.
2 scoops unsweetened whey protein powder	
½ **cup raisins**	
½ **cup dried cranberries**	
½ **cup chopped walnuts**	
⅓ **cup almond milk, per serving**	

Per serving: Calories 255 (From Fat 7); Fat 5.0g (Saturated 0.5g); Cholesterol 1.0mg; Sodium 47mg; Carbohydrate 31g (Dietary Fiber 3g); Protein 6g.

Vary It! For extra flavor, add a splash of orange juice or cranberry juice in addition to the almond milk. And instead of walnuts, substitute ¼ cup sunflower seeds.

Momma Pat's Egg Casserole

Prep time: 20 min, plus refrigeration time • **Cook time:** 50–65 min • **Yield:** 8 servings

Ingredients	Directions
1 pound ground sausage	*1* Butter a 9-x-13-inch baking dish. Preheat the oven to 350 degrees.
Pat of butter to grease baking dish	
5 slices of whole-grain bread, torn into pieces (10–12 ounces)	*2* Brown the sausage in a skillet over medium heat, draining fat as needed.
1½ cups shredded cheddar or colby cheese	*3* Spread the bread crumbles, cheese, and crumbled sausage evenly in a pan.
9 large eggs	
1½ teaspoons dry mustard	*4* In a large bowl, beat the eggs well. Add the mustard and salt and then the milk.
3 cups skim milk	
	5 Pour the mixture over the dry ingredients in the pan and refrigerate overnight.
	6 Bake 45 to 60 minutes, or until the entire casserole is puffed all over.
	7 After removing from the oven, allow the casserole to rest for 5 minutes before serving.

Per serving: Calories 483 (From Fat 180); Fat 20g (Saturated 13g); Cholesterol 233mg; Sodium 594mg; Carbohydrate 19g (Dietary Fiber 4g); Protein 23g.

Tip: Buy eggs from pasture-fed chickens from a local farmer who can guarantee that you're getting chemical-free eggs. Eggs from the grocery store (even the organic ones) are often treated with petroleum mineral oils, chlorine, or other detergents and sanitizers. Every state has its own laws for egg treatments. The U.S. Food and Drug Administration (FDA) "does not have any published regulations dealing with eggshell cleaning and destaining compounds."

Sausage Hash Browns

Prep time: 20 min • **Cook time:** 15 min • **Yield:** 4 servings

Ingredients	*Directions*
½ pound ground sausage	*1* Cook the sausage in a skillet over medium heat until browned, about 8 minutes. Drain fat from skillet as needed.
2 medium Yukon gold or russet potatoes, scrubbed clean	*2* Shred the potatoes, and pat them dry with paper towels.
½ medium onion, diced	
¼ cup whole-wheat flour	*3* In a medium bowl, mix the potatoes, onion, flour, and egg.
1 large egg	
Canola oil	*4* Cover the bottom of a large skillet with approximately ¼ inch of canola oil and heat over medium-high heat.
Salt and ground black pepper to taste	
	5 When the oil is hot, add a ½-inch layer of the shredded potato mixture. Cook until browned on the bottom, approximately 5 to 7 minutes.
	6 Flip the hash browns (use your spatula to divide them into pieces for easier flipping). Sprinkle the browned sausage on top and season with salt and pepper to taste.
	7 Cook another 5 to 7 minutes, until the bottom side is browned.
	8 Serve hot. Pat with paper towels if needed to absorb excess oil.

Per serving: Calories 326 (From Fat 70); Fat 10g (Saturated 7g); Cholesterol 46mg; Sodium 143mg; Carbohydrate 20g (Dietary Fiber 1g); Protein 7g.

Vary It! Add ¼ cup finely shredded cheddar cheese to the potato mixture in Step 3.

Breakfast Quinoa

Prep time: 10 min • **Cook time:** 20 min • **Yield:** 4 servings

Ingredients	*Directions*
2 cups skim milk	*1* Pour the milk into a medium saucepan. Add the quinoa, salt, and cinnamon, and bring to a boil, stirring occasionally.
1 cup organic quinoa	
½ teaspoon salt	
1 teaspoon ground cinnamon	*2* Reduce the heat to low, cover, and simmer for 15 minutes.
1 teaspoon vanilla extract	
5 pitted figs, chopped	*3* When the quinoa is plumped, remove it from the heat.
¼ cup chopped roasted almonds	
	4 Stir in the vanilla, figs, and almonds. Serve warm.

Per serving: Calories 203 (From Fat 52); Fat 6g (Saturated 0.5g); Cholesterol 2.5mg; Sodium 389mg; Carbohydrate 30g (Dietary Fiber 4.5g); Protein 9g.

Vary It! For added flavor, add a drizzle of local honey or 1 tablespoon of organic butter to Step 4.

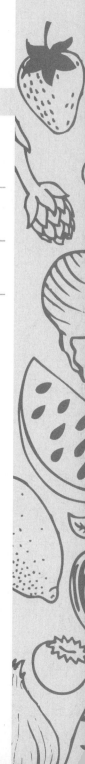

Egg Tacos

Prep time: 15 min • **Cook time:** 5 min • **Yield:** 8 servings

Ingredients	*Directions*
4 large eggs Splash of skim milk ¼ cup diced green onions 8 corn taco shells 1 tablespoon butter 4 tablespoons sour cream ½ cup shredded cheddar or jack cheese 1 tomato, chopped 1 avocado, chopped (optional)	*1* In a medium bowl, crack the eggs and add a splash of milk. Beat well and then add the chopped onions. *2* Heat the taco shells in a toaster oven or a microwave until slightly warm. *3* In a medium skillet, melt the butter over medium heat and then add the egg mixture. *4* Scramble the eggs in the skillet, mixing almost constantly. Cook 3 to 4 minutes, until the eggs are thickened but still moist. Don't overcook. *5* Remove the eggs from the heat immediately and place them in a clean bowl. *6* Coat the inside of each taco shell with sour cream to taste. Spoon approximately 2 tablespoons of egg and 1 tablespoon of cheese into each shell. Add the tomato and avocado (if desired) to taste.

Per serving: Calories 161 (From Fat 95); Fat 11g (Saturated 4g); Cholesterol 113mg; Sodium 258mg; Carbohydrate 11g (Dietary Fiber 1.5g); Protein 7g.

Vary It! For a little extra zing, add a dash of hot sauce to your taco or substitute diced jalapeños for the green onions.

Vegetable Frittata

Prep time: 15 min • **Cook time:** 30 min • **Yield:** 8 servings

Ingredients	Directions
Canola oil no-stick spray	**1** Preheat the oven to 350 degrees. Coat a 9-x-12-inch cake pan or glass baking dish with canola oil no-stick spray. Make sure it's well-coated or the frittata will be difficult to get out of the pan.
2 dozen large eggs	
¼ cup skim milk	
Juice of 1 lemon	**2** In a large bowl, whisk together 8 whole eggs, 16 egg whites, milk, and lemon juice.
Olive oil	
1 cup diced bell peppers (mix red, green, and yellow)	**3** Coat a large sauté pan with olive oil and heat over medium-high heat. Sauté the mixed peppers, spinach, and onion for 3 to 4 minutes, stirring often. Add the mushrooms and mix thoroughly. Salt and pepper to taste, and sauté until the peppers are tender, about 3 more minutes. Remove from the heat and drain off any remaining water or oil.
2 cups fresh spinach	
½ cup diced red onion	
1 cup diced mushrooms (any variety)	
Salt and ground black pepper	**4** Add the vegetables and cheese to the egg mix and stir. Pour the mixture into the cake pan. Sprinkle with salt and pepper.
1 cup shredded cheddar cheese	
	5 Bake 20 to 30 minutes, until the eggs are cooked and the cheese is melted. This dish is delicious hot or cold.

Per serving: Calories 391 (From Fat 250); Fat 28g (Saturated 9g); Cholesterol 568mg; Sodium 438mg; Carbohydrate 9g (Dietary Fiber 1.5g); Protein 25g.

Vary It! Use ¾ cup crumbled feta cheese or goat cheese instead of cheddar.

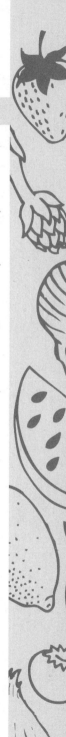

High-Protein Oatmeal

Prep time: 5 min • **Cook time:** 10 min • **Yield:** 2 servings

Ingredients	Directions
Pinch of sea salt	**1** In a medium saucepan, add the salt to the water and bring to a boil over high heat.
2 cups water	
2 cups old-fashioned oats	**2** Add the oatmeal and reduce the heat to medium. Cook for approximately 5 minutes (until all the water is absorbed), stirring frequently.
2 scoops unsweetened whey protein powder (40 grams)	
¼ cup skim milk	**3** Cover and remove from heat. Let stand 1 to 2 minutes.
½ teaspoon ground cinnamon	
½ cup chopped walnuts	**4** In a large bowl, combine the cooked oats, whey powder, milk, cinnamon, and walnuts. Mix thoroughly.
½ ripe banana	
	5 Serve in two large bowls, topped with banana slices. (If the milk cools down the oatmeal, microwave each bowl for 30 seconds before serving.)

Per serving: Calories 455 (From Fat 218); Fat 24g (Saturated 3g); Cholesterol 11mg; Sodium 46mg; Carbohydrate 41g (Dietary Fiber 8g); Protein 15g.

Vary It! Add a handful of raisins or dried cranberries to Step 4.

Chapter 14

Powerful Lunches

In This Chapter

▶ Bringing your lunch to work

▶ Making some tasty and nutritious lunch recipes

*O*ften, lunch is the make-or-break meal that determines what you'll feel like during the rest of the day. Poor choices at lunch leave you with low energy for the afternoon and an unstoppable appetite by the time dinner rolls around.

Under-eating during the day is one of the primary triggers for sugar cravings at night. Be sure that your daytime meals contain lots of protein and fiber to help keep you satiated and energized for the afternoon.

A low-sugar lunch doesn't have to be a dreary sandwich or salad! Instead, use lunch as an opportunity to experience new and exciting foods. In this chapter, I provide some unconventional low-sugar lunch recipes featuring lamb, bison, quinoa, edamame, and loads of fresh, colorful vegetables. Using these examples, you can experiment with some new flavors and textures and make lunchtime a culinary adventure to spice up your day.

Thirst is one of the things that can trigger a sugar craving. Use lunchtime as a reminder to evaluate how much water you've had thus far in the day. Halfway through the day, you should have consumed at least a quart (32 ounces) of water.

Brown-Bagging Tips

If you're not at home during the day, bringing your lunch (and sugar-free snacks) is the only way to ensure that you're supplied with healthy food throughout the day. Here are some tips for planning and packing your lunch:

- ✔ **Plan ahead.** When cooking fish, poultry, or meat for dinner, make some extra for a sandwich or salad for lunch the next day.

- ✔ **Pack a cooler.** If you don't have access to a refrigerator at work (or if you spend your day in the car), stock a cooler with healthy food each morning.

- ✔ **Create an assembly line.** If you're the family's head chef, responsible for making many brown bag lunches in the morning, use the speedy assembly line method:

  1. **Lay out all the slices of bread or wraps in a row.**

  2. **Spread each slice with mustard, hummus, or other low-sugar condiments of your choice.**

     Experiment with spreads like pesto or salsa to make an otherwise uninspired brown-bag sandwich more interesting.

  3. **Go down the line with one ingredient on all slices. Repeat this step for vegetables, cheese, and any other ingredients.**

  4. **Top the sandwiches with the second slice of bread, or roll up wraps.**

  5. **Bag each lunch with love.**

- ✔ **If you'll need to heat your food, pack it in glass containers, not plastic.** When plastics get heated, chemicals like *diethylhexyl adipate, phthalates,* and *bisphenol-a* (BPA) leach out of the plastic. Although the chemicals released from plastics labeled as "microwave safe" are reported to be a tiny, "safe" amount, these chemicals are proven carcinogens and endocrine disruptors. I suggest you don't expose yourself or your family to them if you don't have to.

- ✔ **Start a lunchbox club.** If several of your co-workers or friends bring their own lunches, start a lunchbox club to save everyone time. Assign a day of the week to each person, and on that day he or she will bring a low-sugar lunch for everyone in the group.

Tuna-Stuffed Tomatoes

Prep time: 10 min • **Cook time:** 8–10 min • **Yield:** 2 servings

Ingredients	*Directions*
5-ounce can low-sodium light tuna in water	*1* Preheat the oven or toaster oven to 350 degrees.
2 tablespoons chopped cucumber	*2* Drain the tuna and combine it with the cucumber, onion, celery, olive oil, mayonnaise, lemon juice, and herbs in a medium bowl. Salt and pepper to taste, and stir together thoroughly with a spoon.
2 tablespoons chopped red onion	
2 tablespoons chopped celery	*3* Cut the tomatoes in half horizontally. With a paring knife and spoon, core the tomatoes by scooping out approximately 75 percent of the insides. Discard the tomato innards.
1 tablespoon olive oil	
2 tablespoons mayonnaise	
1 teaspoon fresh-squeezed lemon juice	*4* Fill the cored tomatoes with tuna salad and place them on a baking sheet. Heat them in the oven for 8 to 10 minutes, until the tomatoes are tender and the tuna is warm.
1 teaspoon chopped fresh parsley	
1 teaspoon chopped fresh dill (optional)	
Salt and ground black pepper to taste	
2 large tomatoes	

Per serving: Calories 199 (From Fat 13); Fat 6g (Saturated 1g); Cholesterol 15mg; Sodium 95mg; Carbohydrate 3g (Dietary Fiber 1g); Protein 6g.

Vary It! Add a sprinkling of grated Parmesan cheese to each stuffed tomato before heating.

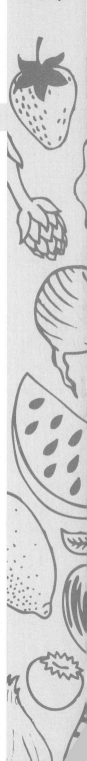

Quinoa and Edamame Salad

Prep time: 10 min • **Cook time:** 25 min • **Yield:** 3–4 servings

Ingredients	*Directions*
2 cups vegetable broth	*1* Rinse the quinoa in a sieve or fine strainer. Toast the quinoa in a dry skillet over medium heat for 5 to 10 minutes, stirring often. Remove from heat when the quinoa begins to crackle.
1 cup quinoa	
2 cups (about 10 ounces) frozen shelled edamame, thawed	*2* After the quinoa toasts approximately 5 minutes, pour the vegetable broth into a large saucepan or small stockpot and bring it to a boil over high heat.
1 cup chopped fresh mushrooms	
1 lemon	*3* Add the quinoa to the boiling broth and return it to a boil. Cover, reduce heat, and simmer for about 8 minutes (the quinoa won't be fully cooked).
2 tablespoons chopped fresh tarragon (or 2 teaspoons dried)	
2 tablespoons olive oil	*4* Add the edamame and mushrooms. Cover and cook for 8 minutes longer, until the edamame and quinoa are tender.
Salt and ground black pepper to taste	
¼ cup chopped walnuts	*5* Halve the lemon and squeeze juice from one half (about 2 tablespoons) into a small bowl. Add the tarragon, olive oil, salt, and pepper, and whisk together.
2 cups fresh spinach or bibb lettuce	
	6 Pour the lemon seasoning mix into the quinoa pot and add the walnuts. Mix thoroughly with a fork.
	7 Plate each salad with a bed of spinach or lettuce. Scoop the edamame/quinoa mix onto each bed.

Per serving: Calories 390 (From Fat 12); Fat 3.5g (Saturated 0.5g); Cholesterol 0mg; Sodium 44mg; Carbohydrate 12g (Dietary Fiber 2.5g); Protein 5g.

Note: This salad is delicious warm or cold.

Vary It! If you're not a fan of edamame, substitute frozen peas or lima beans.

Chicken Broccoli Salad

Prep time: 10 min plus refrigeration time • **Cook time:** 10 min • **Yield:** 4 servings

Ingredients	*Directions*
2 teaspoons olive oil	*1* Coat a small skillet with olive oil and heat it over medium-high heat.
1 boneless, skinless chicken breast (4 to 6 ounces)	*2* Chop the chicken breast into bite-sized pieces and sauté them until browned, about 10 minutes. Stir often.
¼ cup apple cider vinegar	
¾ cup mayonnaise	*3* In a small bowl, whisk the vinegar and mayonnaise together until well blended.
3 cups chopped broccoli florets	
¼ cup chopped walnuts	*4* In a large bowl, mix the broccoli, walnuts, carrots, apple, and cranberries.
1 cup shredded carrots	
½ Fuji apple, cored and chopped	*5* Pour the mayonnaise mix over the broccoli mix. Salt and pepper to taste and toss well.
¼ cup dried cranberries (no added sugar)	*6* Add the chicken and toss again.
Salt and ground black pepper to taste	*7* Refrigerate at least 30 minutes and serve cold.

Per serving: Calories 263 (From Fat 18); Fat 8g (Saturated 1.5g); Cholesterol 16mg; Sodium 147mg; Carbohydrate 8g (Dietary Fiber 2g); Protein 4g.

Vary It! Sauté the chicken in ½ teaspoon curry powder.

Vary It! For a less-crunchy variation, use steamed broccoli instead of raw.

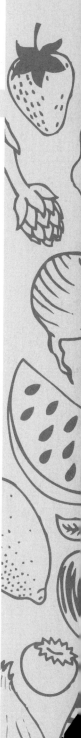

Almond Chicken Salad

Prep time: 5 min • **Yield:** 4 servings

Ingredients	*Directions*
2 cooked boneless, skinless chicken breasts (about 10 ounces combined)	***1*** Chop the cooked chicken breasts into bite-sized pieces.
⅓ cup almond slivers	***2*** In a large bowl, mix the chicken, almonds, grape halves, onion, celery, tarragon, and mayonnaise. Salt and pepper to taste.
½ cup halved red grapes	
1 tablespoon chopped red onion	***3*** Halve the lime and squeeze in lime juice. Mix thoroughly.
1 tablespoon chopped celery	
½ teaspoon tarragon	***4*** Refrigerate or serve immediately on pita bread or Melba toast.
½ cup mayonnaise	
1 fresh lime	
Salt and ground black pepper to taste	
4 pita halves or 8 slices plain Melba toast	

Per serving: Calories 358 (From Fat 17); Fat 10g (Saturated 1.5g); Cholesterol 36mg; Sodium 410mg; Carbohydrate 15g (Dietary Fiber 1.5g); Protein 26g.

Vary 1t! Use walnuts or pistachios instead of almonds.

Vary 1t! Serve the salad on a bed of mixed greens instead of pita or Melba toast.

Greek Salad with Lamb

Prep time: 10 min • **Cook time:** 12 min • **Yield:** 4 servings

Ingredients	*Directions*
2 teaspoons olive oil 1 pound ground lamb	*1* Very lightly coat a large skillet with olive oil and heat it on medium heat.
Salt and ground black pepper to taste 4 cups mixed greens 1 cup cherry tomatoes	*2* Brown the ground lamb in the skillet, breaking it up as it cooks, about 8 to 12 minutes. Remove from heat and drain off excess grease. Add salt and pepper to taste.
1 medium cucumber, washed and sliced 1 cup kalamata olives 1 cup feta cheese	*3* In a large bowl, combine the greens, tomatoes, cucumber, olives, feta, oregano, and lemon juice. Add the olive oil and vinegar, and salt and pepper to taste. Mix well.
1 teaspoon chopped fresh oregano 1 tablespoon fresh lemon juice	*4* Split the salad mix into four plates and divide the ground lamb among the plates. Add a few slices of red onion on top and serve.
1 to 2 teaspoons red wine vinegar, or to taste ½ red onion	

Per serving: Calories 485 (From Fat 35); Fat 12g (Saturated 5g); Cholesterol 50mg; Sodium 192mg; Carbohydrate 3.5g (Dietary Fiber 0.5g); Protein 12g.

Vary It! For a vegetarian option, substitute 2 cups of garbanzo beans (drained and rinsed) for the ground lamb.

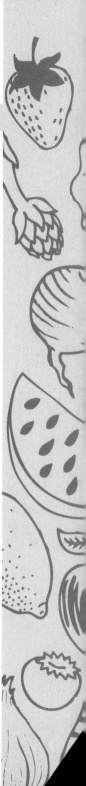

Vegetarian Wraps

Prep time: 10 min • **Cook time:** 10 min • **Yield:** 2 wraps

Ingredients	*Directions*
2 teaspoons olive oil	**1** In a medium skillet, sauté the mushrooms in olive oil over medium-high heat. After 2 minutes, add the bell pepper and continue cooking, stirring often.
2 cups chopped mushrooms	
1 medium red bell pepper, cored and sliced	
Salt and ground black pepper to taste	**2** After about 3 to 5 more minutes, when the pepper starts to soften, add the beans to the skillet to warm them for 3 to 4 more minutes. Stir often.
1 cup cooked garbanzo beans or kidney beans	**3** When the skillet veggies are fully cooked (about 10 minutes total), remove the skillet from the heat. Squeeze lemon juice over the veggies. Add salt and pepper to taste.
½ fresh lemon	
2 large whole-wheat tortillas	**4** Microwave the tortillas for a few seconds to make them easier to wrap and less likely to break. Lay the warm tortillas flat and cover them with the greens, avocado, and tomato. Leave a 1-inch border around the tortilla uncovered.
2 cups fresh spinach or mixed greens	
¼ avocado, chopped	
1 medium tomato, chopped	
	5 Top the tortillas with the warm veggie mix. Wrap them carefully and serve or bag.

Per serving: Calories 498 (From Fat 15); Fat 3g (Saturated 1g); Cholesterol 0mg; Sodium 239mg; Carbohydrate 16g (Dietary Fiber 9g); Protein 5g.

Making smart lunch choices

If you eat a high-protein lunch with lots of organic vegetables, you'll likely stay satisfied, energized, and craving-free for the rest of the day.

Lunches that contain mostly high-glycemic carbs — lots of bread, pasta, or sugar — lead to a sleepy, brain-fogged afternoon. A high-insulin afternoon makes you feel lousy, increases your fat storage, and makes you crave carbs later in the day. Cut back on lunchtime carbs by choosing meals like a mixed green salad with grilled chicken instead of a chicken pasta dish. Using lettuce or kale as the top piece of sandwich bread halves the amount of bread and gives you extra leafy greens to boot.

Use lunch as an opportunity to increase the amount of vegetables in your diet. Load up your sandwich with extra lettuce, tomato, onion, peppers, spinach, olives, mushrooms, or whatever other veggies you like.

Mango Turkey Pitas

Prep time: 15 min • **Cook time:** 10 min • **Yield:** 4–6 servings

Ingredients	*Directions*
1 teaspoon olive oil	*1* Heat the olive oil in a large skillet over medium-high heat.
1 pound ground turkey	
2 teaspoons curry powder	*2* Add the ground turkey, curry powder, and garlic to the skillet. Break up the meat and mix the ingredients as it cooks.
1 teaspoon minced garlic	
Salt and ground black pepper to taste	
1 fresh mango, peeled and chopped	*3* After approximately 4 minutes (the turkey will be white but still juicy), add the mango and tomato to the skillet and reduce the heat to medium. Cook 4 to 5 minutes more, until the turkey is evenly browned and the mango juice has evaporated. Stir often; remove from heat when done. Add salt and pepper to taste.
1 roma tomato, chopped	
2 or 3 whole-wheat pita pockets	
4 tablespoons sour cream	*4* Halve the pita pockets and coat the insides with sour cream. Add a layer of greens.
2 cups mixed greens	
	5 Scoop the turkey mixture into each pocket and serve warm.

Per serving: Calories 289 (From Fat 11); Fat 6g (Saturated 2g); Cholesterol 42mg; Sodium 138mg; Carbohydrate 14g (Dietary Fiber 2g); Protein 14g.

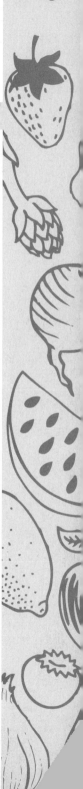

Red Beans and Brown Rice

Prep time: 15 min • **Cook time:** Up to 60 min • **Yield:** 8 servings

Ingredients	*Directions*
4 cups vegetable stock **2 cups brown rice**	*1* In a medium pot, bring the vegetable stock to a boil. Add the rice, cover, and simmer on low heat.
1½ cups canned red beans	*2* Drain and rinse the beans to remove excess salt.
1 large tomato **2 large carrots**	*3* Chop the tomato, carrots, and celery so that they're all the same size.
2 stalks celery **Olive oil** **1 cup diced red onion** **1 tablespoon ground cumin** **1 tablespoon ground coriander**	*4* Coat a medium saucepan in olive oil and combine the onion, carrots, celery, cumin, coriander, and chili powder. Cook 3 to 5 minutes over medium heat, stirring constantly, until the ingredients are browned. Add this into the simmering rice pot.
2 teaspoons chili powder **½ cup fresh or frozen corn kernels** **Garnish: Chopped fresh parsley and/or chopped fresh cilantro**	*5* After approximately 15 minutes, add the beans, tomato, and corn to the rice pot. Continue simmering while covered and continue to stir frequently. Cook the mixture until the stock is absorbed and the rice is fluffy (total cook time varies depending on rice variety).
	6 Remove from heat. Fluff the rice mixture with a fork, top with a sprinkling of parsley and/or cilantro, and serve warm.

Per serving: Calories 158 (From Fat 25); Fat 3g (Saturated 0.5g); Cholesterol 0mg; Sodium 666mg; Carbohydrate 29g (Dietary Fiber 6g); Protein 5g.

Vary It! For more protein, add some diced cooked ham to the vegetables in Step 4.

Dan's No-Bun Big Fun Bison Burgers

Prep time: 10 min • **Cook time:** 12 min • **Yield:** 4 servings

Ingredients	*Directions*
1 pound ground bison	*1* In a large bowl, combine the bison, bread crumbs, mushroom, bell pepper, Worcestershire sauce, and cheese. Mix thoroughly by hand.
½ **cup seasoned panko or Italian bread crumbs**	
½ **cup diced portobello mushroom**	*2* Divide the meat mix into quarters to make four large burger patties approximately ¾- to 1-inch thick.
2 tablespoons diced green bell pepper	
1 tablespoon Worcestershire sauce	*3* Grease a grill or a skillet with olive oil and cook the patties over medium heat, flipping once, until done to preference (5 or 6 minutes per side should do it). Bison cooks better over lower heat and for a longer time compared to beef, and it tastes better when cooked to medium-rare or rare, depending on your preference.
½ **cup grated Parmigiano-Reggiano cheese**	
1 teaspoon olive oil	
1 head organic bibb lettuce	*4* Remove the patties and serve them wrapped in bibb lettuce leaves instead of on a traditional bun. (I recommend at least two pieces of lettuce for each "slice" of bun on the top and bottom.) Add salt and pepper to taste.
½ **teaspoon salt**	
¼ **teaspoon ground black pepper**	

Per serving: Calories 305 (From Fat 14); Fat 5g (Saturated 2.5g); Cholesterol 33mg; Sodium 610mg; Carbohydrate 4g (Dietary Fiber 0.5g); Protein 35g.

Vary It! If you don't have access to ground bison, you can use ground beef instead. If you're using beef, make slightly thinner patties. Cook time may be slightly longer.

Vary It! For spicier burgers, add ½ teaspoon of chopped jalapeños or Cajun spice to Step 1. You can also top the burgers with the cheese of your choice.

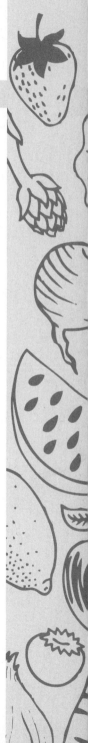

Ostrich Medallions with Corn Relish

Prep time: 15 min • **Cook time:** 15 min • **Yield:** 4 servings

Ingredients	Directions
3 tablespoons plus 1 teaspoon olive oil, divided	**1** Grease an iron skillet with 1 teaspoon of olive oil and heat over medium-high heat.
½ teaspoon paprika	
½ teaspoon dry mustard	**2** In a small bowl, mix 3 tablespoons olive oil, paprika, mustard, cayenne, salt, and pepper. Remove 1 teaspoon of this seasoned oil to add to the corn relish.
¼ teaspoon cayenne pepper	
¼ teaspoon salt	
¼ teaspoon ground black pepper	**3** Brush the ostrich medallions heavily with the remaining seasoned oil.
Eight 2-ounce ostrich medallions	**4** When the skillet is hot, sear the medallions for 2 minutes on one side. Turn them with tongs, cover, and turn off the heat. Allow the medallions to rest in the skillet for 4 to 5 minutes.
Corn Relish (see the following recipe)	
	5 Serve the warm medallions topped with the cold Corn Relish.

Corn Relish

1 cup frozen corn kernels (about 2 ears if fresh)

¼ cup diced red bell pepper

2 tablespoons chopped red onion

2 tablespoons chopped white onion

2 tablespoons chopped celery

¼ cup cider vinegar

1 tablespoon canola oil

Salt and ground black pepper to taste

1 Cook frozen corn according to package instructions. If you're using fresh corn, fill a small saucepan halfway with salted water and bring it to a boil. Add the corn and cook it for approximately 5 minutes, until the corn is tender. Drain and cool the corn under cold running water. Shake off excess water in a strainer. Pat the corn kernels dry.

2 In a medium bowl, mix the corn, bell pepper, red onion, white onion, celery, vinegar, and canola oil. Add the seasoned oil mix that you set aside while preparing the ostrich medallions. Mix well and refrigerate.

Per serving: Calories 314 (From Fat 20); Fat 15g (Saturated 2.5g); Cholesterol 69mg; Sodium 174mg; Carbohydrate 1.5g (Dietary Fiber 0.5g); Protein 22g.

Tip: Garnish the ostrich medallions with dark greens like kale or turnip.

Tip: Ostrich meat contains very little fat, so overcooking it even a little can dry it out quickly. Be sure to pull the medallions out of the skillet while there's still a good bit of red in the centers.

Vary It! If you don't have access to ostrich meat, try this recipe with thin slices of beef. Cooking times for beef may be longer.

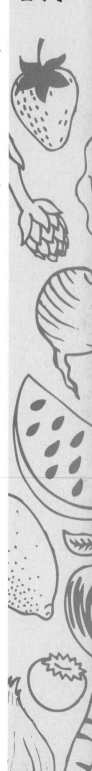

Low-Carb Surf and Turf Sandwich

Prep time: 5 min • **Cook time:** 10 min • **Yield:** 2 servings

Ingredients	*Directions*
4 ounces raw shrimp, shelled and cleaned	*1* Cut the shrimp into bite-sized pieces.
1 teaspoon butter ½ teaspoon green onion or shallot, chopped 1 thumb-sized piece of avocado	*2* Heat the butter in a medium skillet over medium heat until the butter bubbles. Add the shrimp and onions, and cook approximately 2 minutes, until the shrimp is no longer opaque. Stir frequently. If you use shallot instead of green onion, sauté the shallot for 1 minute before adding the shrimp.
Salt and ground black pepper to taste Two 4-ounce cuts of leftover grilled steak or pork loin	*3* Chop the avocado into quarter-inch cubes and mix it with the cooked shrimp and onions. Salt and pepper to taste.
	4 Carefully slice the leftover steak or pork in half horizontally. Heat the meat slices in the microwave for 20 to 30 seconds, or until the meat is warm.
	5 Sandwich the shrimp mix in between two slices of meat, grab a napkin, and enjoy!

Per serving: Calories 334 (From Fat 15); Fat 8g (Saturated 3g); Cholesterol 120mg; Sodium 334mg; Carbohydrate 1g (Dietary Fiber 0.5g); Protein 25g.

Note: If this dish is too messy to eat as a sandwich, eat it with a fork and knife instead.

Vary It! Cook shrimp and onions in the sauce of your choice — Worcestershire, teriyaki, Cajun spices, and so on.

Chapter 15

Nourishing Dinners

In This Chapter

▶ Making healthy dinners quickly

▶ Checking out some speedy dinner recipes

*I*f you're the head chef in your family, dinnertime can be stressful. Not only are you responsible for feeding yourself sensibly, but you also have several other people to consider, each with his or her own tastes, preferences, and sometimes, specific dietary requirements. Not to mention that every day you face the time crunch of trying to create a healthy meal in a hurry after a long day at work!

Pleasing everyone in the family with your low-sugar menu planning can be a challenge. You may very well face some resistance to changing to a healthier eating style; if that's the case, turn to Chapter 9 for some tips on transitioning the family food plan.

Dinnertime isn't just about the food. Often, a few minutes together at the dinner table is the only time family members have to connect with one another. Be sure to appreciate this time together, and use it to listen, learn, and bond.

Whipping Up Speedy Dinner Recipes

One difficulty that lots of clients have expressed to me over the years is finding the time to cook healthy meals. When you work long days and the kids have after-school activities, you don't have a lot of time left for cooking. Here are some tips for cutting down your time in the kitchen:

✔ **Build a repertoire of dependable recipes.** Master a handful of recipes so you can make them without thinking. That way you always have a healthy fallback if you're pressed for time when 6 p.m. rolls around.

How to thaw meat quickly

The best way to thaw frozen meat is not to leave it thawing in the sink but to move it to the refrigerator, where it will thaw evenly in a day or two and stay at a safe temperature the whole time. However, sometimes forgetfulness or a last-minute change of plans requires you to cook something that's still frozen.

Don't defrost meat in the microwave. It heats too unevenly, and you'll have some parts partially cooked and some parts still frozen. The meat won't cook well in the oven or on the stovetop.

Don't run a package of meat under hot (or even warm) water. Doing so starts to cook the meat on the outer edges.

The correct way to thaw frozen meat quickly is to place the package in a bowl filled with cold water and place the bowl under the kitchen faucet with a cold-water drip. Adjust the faucet so you get a tiny stream of water, just slightly faster than being able to count the drips. Rotate the package occasionally.

✔ **Plan your menus several days ahead.** That way you have plenty of time to procure any special ingredients, and when it's time to hit the kitchen, you already know what's going to happen and you're ready to dive in.

✔ **Do the prep for several meals at once.** Plan your meals for a few days at a time, and when you're chopping up stuff for one of them, do the prep work for the next meal or two while you have the cutting board out. Fill storage containers with ingredients ready to grab for the next few times you're cooking.

✔ **Read through the recipe first.** Before you start cooking, make sure you have all the ingredients on hand. To speed the process, look for places you can multi-task while water is boiling or food is cooking.

✔ **Enjoy the process.** Don't panic every time something needs cooked in the kitchen. The children won't perish if dinner isn't ready by 6. Stop stressing yourself out, and enjoy the process of preparing healthy food for your family. They may enjoy getting involved, too!

✔ **Find some organic, low-sugar bottled sauces.** Premade sauces can add some zing to an otherwise uninspiring chicken-and-veggie dish. Experiment with jarred salsa, teriyaki, hoisin, or pesto sauces — the low-sugar kinds, of course!

Honey Dijon Salmon

Prep time: 5 min • **Cook time:** 15–20 min • **Yield:** 4 servings

Ingredients	*Directions*
¼ **cup Dijon mustard**	**1** Preheat the oven to 425 degrees.
2 tablespoons maltitol syrup (sugar-free honey substitute)	**2** Whisk together the mustard, maltitol, and vinegar in a small bowl.
½ **tablespoon red wine vinegar**	
Four 4–5 ounce wild-caught salmon filets	**3** Place the filets in a baking dish and brush them with the mustard mixture. Coat thoroughly.
Salt and ground black pepper to taste	**4** Bake 15 to 20 minutes, depending on the thickness of the filets. Salmon is done when the flesh is whitish pink and flakes with a fork.
	5 Salt and pepper to taste.

Per serving: Calories 262 (From Fat 135); Fat 15g (Saturated 3g); Cholesterol 81mg; Sodium 426mg; Carbohydrate 6g (Dietary Fiber 0g); Protein 28g.

Tip: Serve with a side of steamed asparagus or sautéed spinach.

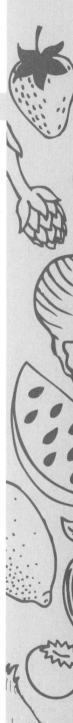

Lemon Caper Tilapia

Prep time: 6 min • **Cook time:** 10–15 min • **Yield:** 4 servings

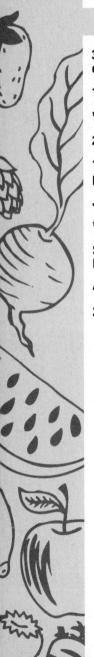

Ingredients	*Directions*
3 tablespoons olive oil, divided	*1* Heat 1 tablespoon of olive oil in a small saucepan over medium heat. When the oil is hot, sauté the shallots for about 1½ minutes.
1 shallot, minced	
½ cup white wine	*2* Add the wine and increase the heat to high. Boil 3 to 5 minutes, until the sauce is reduced to approximately ¼ cup.
2 tablespoons butter	
1 tablespoon chopped fresh parsley	*3* Strain the sauce and discard the shallot pieces. Return the sauce to the pan.
Juice of ½ lemon	
¼ cup rice flour	*4* Whisk in the butter and parsley. Squeeze lemon juice into the mixture and stir briefly (watch out for lemon seeds). Set the sauce aside.
Sprinkle of salt and ground black pepper	
4 large tilapia filets	*5* Heat the remaining 2 tablespoons of olive oil in a large skillet on medium-high heat until it's simmering but not smoking. If the oil smokes, it's too hot and you need to start over with fresh oil.
2 tablespoons capers	
	6 While the oil heats, spread the rice flour on a plate and sprinkle it with salt and pepper.

7	Rinse the tilapia filets in cold water, and then coat both sides of each filet in the rice flour mix.
8	When the oil is heated, place the filets in the skillet and reduce to medium heat.
9	Cook the filets 2 to 3 minutes on one side, until the edges are opaque and the bottoms are browned.
10	Flip the filets and sprinkle the capers on top. Cook on this side 2 to 3 minutes, until the bottom is brown and the thickest part of the filet is soft.
11	Plate each filet and top with the desired amount of sauce. Be sure to get some capers onto each filet.

Per serving: Calories 341 (From Fat 171); Fat 19g (Saturated 6g); Cholesterol 76mg; Sodium 271mg; Carbohydrate 10g (Dietary Fiber 0.5g); Protein 29g.

Tip: Serve tilapia filets over a bed of fresh spinach sautéed in olive oil.

What's the difference between wet scallops and dry scallops?

Wet scallops are commonly treated with phosphates as a preservative. When scallops are soaked in phosphates they absorb water, and this makes them weigh more (and cost you more). The absorbed water evaporates during cooking, leaving the scallops shrunken, dry, and often tasteless. Furthermore, the added water doesn't let scallops brown properly during cooking. Phosphate-treated scallops usually appear snow-white in color.

Dry scallops are all-natural and haven't been treated with any chemicals. They're harvested directly from the ocean, shucked on deck, and immediately frozen on the boat to preserve quality. Dry scallops caramelize during cooking to a golden brown color that's very attractive when served. Raw dry scallops have a natural vanilla color.

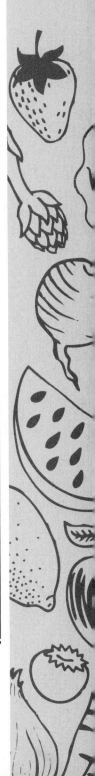

Ginger Scallop Casserole

Prep time: 15 min • **Cook time:** 15 min • **Yield:** 4 servings

Ingredients	*Directions*
2 green onions	*1* Preheat the oven to 400 degrees.
1 small clove garlic	
⅓ cup dry sherry	*2* Finely dice the onions (enough for ¼ cup) and garlic.
3 tablespoons low-sodium soy sauce	*3* Stir together the sherry, soy sauce, sesame oil, ginger, onions, and garlic in a small bowl.
2 teaspoons sesame oil	
1 teaspoon grated fresh ginger	*4* Rinse the scallops in cold water and pat them dry with a paper towel. If the scallops are large, cut them in half through the thickness.
2 pounds dry bay scallops (see sidebar)	
3 tablespoons butter	*5* Place the scallops in a casserole dish. Cut the butter into five or six pieces and scatter throughout the dish. Sprinkle with salt and pepper.
Dash of salt and ground black pepper	
1 cup panko or plain bread crumbs	*6* Pour the ginger sauce over the scallops and butter. Sprinkle the bread crumbs over the scallops.
	7 Bake approximately 15 minutes, until the edges of the scallops are golden and the flesh is slightly firm.

Per serving: Calories 440 (From Fat 118); Fat 13g (Saturated 6g); Cholesterol 116mg; Sodium 2,086mg; Carbohydrate 26g (Dietary Fiber 1g); Protein 49g.

Tip: Serve scallops with wild rice, quinoa, or couscous.

Vary It! This ginger sauce goes well with white fish, too. Try orange roughy, sole, or flounder. You may have to adjust the baking time accordingly.

Coconut Lime Shrimp

Prep time: 8 min • **Cook time:** 35 min • **Yield:** 4 servings

Ingredients	Directions
1 cup basmati rice or quinoa	**1** Boil water and cook the rice or quinoa according to the package instructions.
1 lime	
1 pound uncooked shrimp, peeled and deveined	**2** Zest a small amount of lime on a cheese grater.
Sea salt	**3** In a bowl, add the shrimp, lime zest, and a pinch of salt. Squeeze in the lime juice and let marinate for 15 minutes.
2 teaspoons olive oil	
¾ cup unsweetened coconut milk	**4** In a large skillet, heat the olive oil over medium heat. Sauté the shrimp 1 to 2 minutes and then remove them from the skillet and set them aside.
¼ cup chopped fresh cilantro	
2 tablespoons chopped mint	
4 scallions (both white and green parts), chopped	**5** In the same skillet, combine the coconut milk, cilantro, mint, scallions, and peanuts. Cook 1 minute.
2 tablespoons chopped unsalted roasted peanuts	**6** Stir in the shrimp and cook 1 minute more, stirring constantly.
	7 Serve the shrimp and sauce on a bed of rice or quinoa.

Per serving: Calories 401 (From Fat 148); Fat 16g (Saturated 10g); Cholesterol 143mg; Sodium 352mg; Carbohydrate 44g (Dietary Fiber 2.5g); Protein 21g.

Tip: To add some zing, add a chopped jalapeño pepper to Step 5.

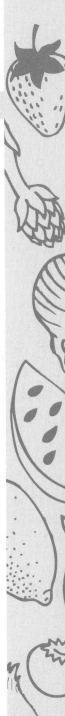

Halibut with Blueberry Mango Salsa

Prep time: 15 min • **Cook time:** 10 min • **Yield:** 4 servings

Ingredients	Directions
2 tablespoons olive oil	**1** Coat a large skillet with olive oil and heat over medium-high heat. Salt and pepper the halibut filets and dust them with cornmeal.
Salt and ground black pepper	
Four 4-ounce halibut filets	
1–2 tablespoons cornmeal	**2** Cook the halibut 3 to 5 minutes on each side, until flaky.
Blueberry Mango Salsa (see the following recipe)	
	3 Serve each halibut filet topped with approximately ¼ cup Blueberry Mango Salsa.

Blueberry Mango Salsa

⅓ cup fresh blueberries	**1** Combine the blueberries, mango, onion, cilantro, and jalapeño in a bowl. Add the lime juice and a pinch of salt.
⅓ cup peeled and diced mango	
2 tablespoons minced red onion	**2** Lightly crush the mixture with the back of a fork until juicy.
1 tablespoon chopped fresh cilantro	
½ teaspoon minced jalapeño pepper	
Juice from ½ lime	
Salt to taste	

Per serving: Calories 221 (From Fat 84); Fat 9g (Saturated 1g); Cholesterol 35mg; Sodium 61mg; Carbohydrate 9g (Dietary Fiber 0.5g); Protein 24g.

Tip: This dish goes well with a warm polenta cake or some sautéed kale.

Vary It! Experiment with different kinds of fish, such as salmon, tuna, or catfish.

Baked Parmesan Chicken

Prep time: 7 min • **Cook time:** 40–50 min • **Yield:** 4 servings

Ingredients	*Directions*
4 boneless, skinless chicken breasts	*1* Preheat the oven to 350 degrees. Grease a 9-x-13-inch baking dish with butter.
½ cup panko or Italian bread crumbs	*2* Rinse the chicken breasts under cold tap water and set them aside.
½ cup freshly grated Parmigiano-Reggiano cheese	*3* Mix the bread crumbs, cheese, Fresh Italian Seasoning, salt, and pepper in a shallow dish.
¼ cup Fresh Italian Seasoning (see the following recipe)	
½ teaspoon salt	*4* Beat the egg in a separate shallow dish.
¼ teaspoon ground black pepper	*5* Dip each chicken breast in the egg, and then press it into the seasoned crumb mix, coating both sides heavily. Place in the baking dish.
1 large egg	
	6 Bake chicken breasts uncovered for 40 to 50 minutes, until internal temperature reads 165 degrees with a meat thermometer.

Fresh Italian Seasoning

2 tablespoons minced fresh basil	*1* Mix all ingredients together in a small bowl.
1 tablespoon minced fresh oregano	
2 tablespoons minced fresh parsley	
1 dime-sized garlic clove, minced	

Per serving: *Calories 281 (From Fat 80); Fat 9g (Saturated 3.5g); Cholesterol 150mg; Sodium 482mg; Carbohydrate 6g (Dietary Fiber 1g); Protein 42g.*

Tip: Because the bake time on this dish is almost an hour, it may work better as a weekend dinner when you're not rushed for time.

Tip: This dish goes well with baked potatoes or roasted red potatoes. It's also excellent with a strong-flavored green like kale or turnip greens.

Chipotle Turkey Medallions

Prep time: 20 min • **Cook time:** 15 min • **Yield:** 4 servings

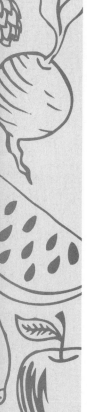

Ingredients	*Directions*
1 pound boneless, skinless turkey breasts	**1** Preheat the oven to 400 degrees.
1 tablespoon local honey or maltitol syrup	**2** Cut the turkey breasts into eight medallions, each 2 inches in diameter. Pound them with a meat mallet until they're ¼ inch thick. If the breast is very thick, you may need to butterfly it (slice almost all the way through the thickness and open it up like butterfly wings) and then pound it thin.
2 tablespoons butter	
¼ teaspoon ground chipotle chile pepper (or more to taste)	
Pinch of salt	
2 cups cubed potatoes (a medley of your choice)	**3** In a small saucepan, warm the honey or maltitol on medium-low heat, taking care not to boil it. Add the butter and stir.
No-stick spray	
1 teaspoon fresh rosemary	**4** When the butter has melted, remove the pan from the heat and stir in the chipotle seasoning and a pinch of salt.
Sprinkle of ground black pepper	
2 tablespoons olive oil	**5** Spread the potato medley on a large baking sheet greased with no-stick spray. Sprinkle with rosemary, salt, and pepper. Roast for approximately 10 minutes, until the potatoes are tender.
	6 While the potatoes are roasting, coat a large skillet with 1 tablespoon olive oil and heat over medium heat. Sauté the turkey medallions 2 to 3 minutes on one side, until golden-brown. Flip the medallions.
	7 Add the honey chipotle sauce to the pan with the turkey medallions and cook 2 to 3 minutes, until the sauce is slightly thick.
	8 Place 2 medallions on each dinner plate and top with about a tablespoon of chipotle sauce. Serve with ½ cup of roasted potato medley drizzled with 1 tablespoon olive oil.

Per serving: Calories 360 (From Fat 153); Fat 17g (Saturated 5g); Cholesterol 96mg; Sodium 182mg; Carbohydrate 15g (Dietary Fiber 1g); Protein 35g.

Tip: Serve with a side of steamed broccoli or a large, mixed green salad.

Grilled Cajun Beef Kebabs

Prep time: 12 min • **Cook time:** 8–9 min • **Yield:** 4 servings

Ingredients	*Directions*
8 wooden skewers	**1** Soak the wooden skewers in warm water for 20 to 30 minutes. Preheat a charcoal or gas grill.
1 large green bell pepper	
12 cherry tomatoes	**2** Wash all the vegetables and cut everything except the cherry tomatoes into squares approximately 1-x-1-inch.
1 purple onion	
1 large portobello mushroom	**3** Cut the beef into 1-inch cubes and dip them into the basting sauce.
8 ounces beef filet (or beef tips)	
Cajun Basting Sauce (see the following recipe)	**4** Alternate skewering pieces of pepper, tomato, beef, onion, and mushroom onto skewers until they're full.
Salt and ground black pepper	**5** Heavily brush the kebabs with the Cajun Basting Sauce. Sprinkle the kebabs with salt and pepper.
	6 Brush the grill with olive oil. Grill the kebabs with the grill lid closed, until the edges of the meat and vegetables are crispy (approximately 8 to 9 minutes), using tongs to turn the skewers frequently.

Cajun Basting Sauce

¼ cup olive oil	**1** Whisk together all ingredients in a small bowl.
Juice of 1 lime	
1 teaspoon minced fresh oregano	
2 tablespoons Cajun spice	
1 teaspoon Worcestershire sauce	

Per serving: Calories 303 (From Fat 227); Fat 34g (Saturated 6g); Cholesterol 39mg; Sodium 53mg; Carbohydrate 9g (Dietary Fiber 1.5g); Protein 13g.

Vary It! Serve mini-kebabs as an appetizer or use them as a snack to take to work. On a short skewer, slide one piece of beef in between two vegetables.

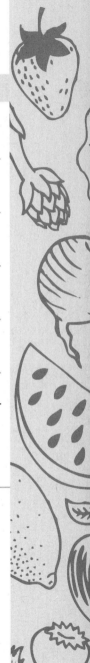

Lamb Pockets

Prep time: 25 min, plus refrigeration time • **Cook time:** 12 min • **Yield:** 4–6 pockets

Ingredients	Directions
1 pound ground lamb	**1** Brown the ground lamb in a skillet over medium heat, stirring often. Don't overcook. Add spices to taste.
2 teaspoons red curry powder or ground cumin	
2 tablespoons minced red onion	**2** When the lamb is approximately halfway cooked (about 4 minutes), sprinkle the red onion into the skillet.
4 whole-wheat pita pockets	
Tzatziki Sauce (see the following recipe)	**3** Slice the pita circles in half. Stir the refrigerated Tzatziki Sauce with a spoon and coat the insides of the pita pockets.
Handful of fresh lettuce	
Handful of fresh spinach	**4** Line the pockets with fresh lettuce and spinach to taste.
	5 When the lamb is fully cooked, scoop a 4-ounce serving into a separate bowl. Add a teaspoon (or more, if you like) of Tzatziki Sauce and mix.
	6 Stuff the sauced lamb into the pockets and serve hot.

Tzatziki Sauce

2 medium cucumbers	*1* Peel the cucumbers and cut them in half lengthwise. Scoop out the seeds with a spoon.
½ teaspoon sea salt	
1 small clove garlic, minced	*2* Dice the cucumbers and press them dry with a paper towel. Sprinkle with salt.
Juice of 1 lemon	
Ground black pepper	*3* Place the salted cucumber, garlic, lemon juice, and a few grinds of black pepper in a blender or food processor and process on medium speed until well blended.
3 cups Greek yogurt	
1 tablespoon chopped fresh dill	*4* Stir this mix into the Greek yogurt. Add the dill and stir thoroughly. Refrigerate, preferably for several hours to allow the flavors to blend. You'll need to re-stir the sauce every time you use it.

Per serving: Calories 478 (From Fat 205); Fat 23g (Saturated 10g); Cholesterol 66mg; Sodium 730mg; Carbohydrate 35g (Dietary Fiber 5g); Protein 34g.

Tip: Although the hot lamb contrasted with the cold cucumber is appealing to some, you may want to microwave the assembled pocket for 15 seconds if you prefer it warm.

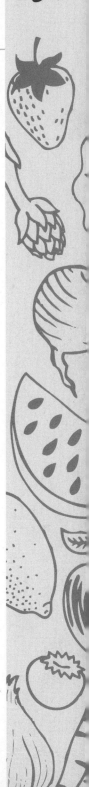

Vegetarian Pasta Pomodoro

Prep time: 8 min • **Cook time:** 25 min • **Yield:** 4 servings

Ingredients	*Directions*
Pomodoro Sauce (see the following recipe)	*1* Prepare the Pomodoro Sauce.
Sea salt	*2* Boil 5 to 6 cups of salted water in a large saucepan. While the water is heating, wash and chop the zucchini, squash, and mushrooms.
5–6 cups water	
1 small zucchini	
1 small yellow squash	*3* Add the rice pasta to the boiling water and cook approximately 8 minutes, stirring occasionally.
½ cup chopped mushrooms of your choice	
8 ounces brown rice spaghetti	*4* While the pasta cooks, sauté the zucchini, squash, and mushrooms in a small saucepan with olive oil.
2 tablespoons olive oil	
	5 When the pasta reaches desired doneness, drain it and serve it topped with vegetables and Pomodoro Sauce.

Pomodoro Sauce

1 carrot	**1** Dice the carrot and celery, and mince the garlic.
1 celery stalk	
1 clove garlic	**2** Lightly coat a medium sauté pan with olive oil, and sauté the carrot, celery, and garlic over medium heat until golden. Add salt.
¼ teaspoon salt	
15-ounce can diced tomatoes	
2 tablespoons olive oil	**3** Add the diced tomatoes, olive oil, bay leaf, and vegetable broth. Stir in the tomato paste.
1 bay leaf	
¼ cup vegetable broth	**4** Simmer (barely) for 15 to 20 minutes, stirring occasionally. Do not boil!
½ cup tomato paste	
1 tablespoon chopped fresh basil	**5** Before serving, remove the bay leaf. Sprinkle with basil and oregano when serving.
1 teaspoon chopped fresh oregano	

Per serving: Calories 228 (From Fat 101); Fat 11g (Saturated 2.5g); Cholesterol 19mg; Sodium 1,383mg; Carbohydrate 28g (Dietary Fiber 4.5g); Protein 7g.

Vary It! You can use any pasta you like with this sauce. Rice pasta is wheat-free and gluten-free and doesn't tend to get as mushy as semolina pasta. It's high in fiber too!

Vary It! Nonvegetarians who want more protein in this dish can add 6 to 8 ounces of sautéed chicken or pork.

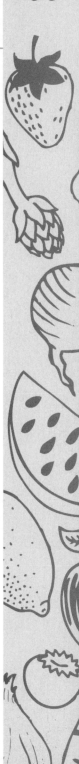

Chapter 16

Satisfying Snacks

In This Chapter

▶ Choosing snacks that add nutrition to your diet

▶ Whipping up some healthy and delicious snacks

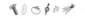
*H*ealthy snacks are crucial for keeping your blood sugar levels steady and for fending off sugar cravings. The right snacks satisfy your hunger and fuel your body for a few hours, leaving you sharp, energetic, and craving-free. The wrong snacks (or no snacks at all) cause that familiar midafternoon sinking feeling, which triggers a drive for something sweet.

Many of the snack recipes in this chapter are designed to be prepared and portioned out in advance so that they're easy to grab when you need a healthy snack in a hurry. Herein you find a high-protein apple walnut loaf, nutritious veggie burgers, tasty shrimp salad, and delicious protein bars that will be ready to go when you are!

Understanding Snacking Success

When planning your snacks, think of them as mini-meals. Using the same nutrition principles you use with breakfast, lunch, and dinner, make sure your snacks contain a protein and a plant (see Chapter 5), and plan out your snack times in your schedule so you're sure to supply yourself with healthy nutrition during the day.

Healthy snacks add quality nutrition to your daily diet. Use your prepared snacks as an opportunity to put more vitamins, minerals, protein, and antioxidants into your body. Grabbing something from a vending machine or from the candy jar just adds extra calories without any worthwhile nutrients.

Plan ahead! If you leave the house without knowing what you're going to eat throughout the day, you leave yourself at the mercy of whatever is lying around in the break room at work, or whatever you can grab at a drive-through restaurant. Be smart and purposeful in your food planning so you can avoid reactive eating and stay a step ahead of those pesky sugar cravings!

Need a snack in a pinch? Eggs to the rescue!

A hard-boiled egg can be your go-to snack if you have zero time to get something healthy to eat. Downing an egg or two quells your hunger, adds extra protein for the day, and keeps your starving brain from driving you to sugar.

A common problem with hard-boiling eggs is that you can easily overcook them, leading to a dark green tint around the yolk and a sulfur taste. To boil eggs without overcooking, place a dozen pasture-fed eggs in a saucepan and add cold water until the top of the water line is two inches above the eggs. To keep the eggs from cracking, salt the water and gradually bring it to a boil. When the water is boiling, reduce the heat and simmer for about a minute. Then remove the pan from the burner, cover, and let sit for 12 minutes. Extra-large eggs need a few minutes more (15 to 17 minutes). If you're

cooking a half-dozen eggs, you can cut the time to 9 minutes.

Remove the eggs with a slotted spoon and place them into a bowl of ice water. After they cool, strain the water from the eggs and refrigerate them in a covered container to protect your refrigerator from a strong egg odor. Eggs that have been refrigerated for a few days peel easier than fresher eggs.

One way to test whether your eggs are fully cooked is to set the larger end of the boiled egg on a hard surface, like a countertop or a table. Spin the egg the same way you would spin a top. A hard-boiled egg spins evenly and swiftly because the yolk is solid. An egg with an undercooked yolk doesn't spin well; it wobbles around instead of spinning in one spot.

Apple Cinnamon Walnut Loaf

Prep time: 10 min • **Cook time:** 50–60 min • **Yield:** 12 servings

Ingredients	*Directions*
3 tablespoons skim milk	*1* Preheat the oven to 350 degrees. Grease and flour a 9-x-5-inch loaf pan.
6 tablespoons softened butter	
2 tablespoons local honey	*2* Mix the milk, butter, and honey in a medium bowl with an electric mixer on medium speed until the mix is light and fluffy. Gradually add the eggs and whey powder while continuing to beat.
2 eggs	
1 scoop (20 grams or 4 teaspoons) whey protein powder (vanilla or unflavored)	
1¾ cups all-purpose flour	*3* In a separate bowl, whisk together the flour, baking powder, salt, and baking soda. Stir this mix into the butter/egg batter until it's blended.
1 teaspoon baking powder	
½ teaspoon salt	*4* Stir in the applesauce, cinnamon, and walnuts until blended.
½ teaspoon baking soda	
1 cup unsweetened applesauce	*5* Pour the batter into the loaf pan and bake for 50 to 60 minutes, until a toothpick inserted into the center comes out clean.
1 teaspoon ground cinnamon	
6 ounces walnuts, chopped	*6* Remove the loaf from the oven and cool it in the pan on a wire rack for 10 minutes. Remove the loaf from the pan and finish cooling it on the rack. Store at room temperature wrapped in foil.

Per serving: Calories 252 (From Fat 148); Fat 16g (Saturated 5g); Cholesterol 50mg; Sodium 454mg; Carbohydrate 21g (Dietary Fiber 2g); Protein 7g.

Vary It! Add ¼ cup raisins to Step 4.

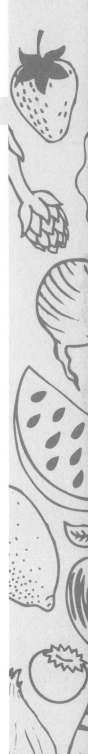

Chocolate Peanut Butter Protein Bars

Prep time: 10 min • **Cook time:** 5 min • **Yield:** 24 bars

Ingredients	*Directions*
1 cup creamy peanut butter	**1** In a glass bowl, stir together the peanut butter and honey. Microwave for 60 seconds, until the mixture stirs easily.
¼ cup local honey	
1 cup whey protein powder (vanilla or unflavored)	**2** In a separate bowl, blend together the protein powder, oats, almond meal, and cocoa powder.
½ cup slow-cook oats	
¾ cup almond meal	**3** Add the protein mix to the peanut butter and honey and mix thoroughly (it will be very thick).
2 tablespoons cocoa powder	
3 ounces dark chocolate (70% cacao)	**4** Press the mixture into a 9-x-16-inch baking pan, approximately 1 inch thick. Optionally, roll the mixture into balls instead.
	5 Place the baking pan in the freezer for 5 to 10 minutes, until the mix starts to harden a little.
	6 In a medium saucepan, slowly melt the chocolate. When the chocolate is melted, remove the pan from the freezer and coat the mix with the melted chocolate.
	7 Return the pan to the freezer; remove it when the chocolate hardens.
	8 Cut into 24 servings. Serve at room temperature.

Per serving: Calories 149 (From Fat 84); Fat 9g (Saturated 2.5g); Cholesterol 17mg; Sodium 67mg; Carbohydrate 8g (Dietary Fiber 1.5g); Protein 10g.

Vary It! Add ¼ cup coconut or pecan pieces to Step 2.

Three Bean Quinoa Salad

Prep time: 5 min • **Cook time:** 25 min • **Yield:** 6 servings

Ingredients	Directions
2 cups water	*1* In a medium saucepan, bring the water to a boil. Add the quinoa, cover, and reduce the heat. Simmer for approximately 20 minutes, until the water is absorbed. Remove from the heat and fluff the quinoa with a fork.
1 cup quinoa	
One 15-ounce can black beans, drained and rinsed	
One 15-ounce can red beans, drained and rinsed	*2* Mix in the beans, olive oil, vinegar, and Italian seasoning. Stir well. Salt and pepper to taste.
One 15-ounce can white beans, drained and rinsed	
¼ cup olive oil	*3* Refrigerate for at least two hours before serving.
¼ cup red wine vinegar	
2 teaspoons Italian seasoning	
Salt and ground black pepper to taste	

Per serving: Calories 296 (From Fat 90); Fat 10g (Saturated 1.5g); Cholesterol 0mg; Sodium 458mg; Carbohydrate 42g (Dietary Fiber 11g); Protein 13g.

Vary It! Add ½ cup chopped roasted red peppers or chopped kalamata olives to Step 2.

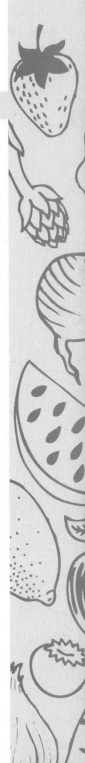

Chicken Broccoli Taters

Prep time: 10 min • **Cook time:** 45 min • **Yield:** 4 servings

Ingredients	Directions
2 medium russet potatoes Olive oil One 4-ounce boneless skinless chicken breast Cajun spice to taste Salt and ground black pepper to taste 1 cup broccoli, chopped ¼ cup shredded sharp cheddar or jack cheese Sour cream or fresh salsa for serving	**1** Preheat the oven to 400 degrees. Wash the potatoes thoroughly, wrap them in foil, vent each with a fork five times, and place them on a cookie sheet or directly onto the oven rack. Bake for 45 minutes. To test doneness, poke one with a knife to check for tenderness — a cooked potato is soft throughout, so cook them longer if they're still firm inside. **2** While the potatoes bake, coat a medium skillet with olive oil and heat over medium-high heat. **3** Chop the chicken breast into bite-sized pieces and cook them in the skillet, stirring often. Add the Cajun spice, salt, and pepper to taste. **4** When the chicken is no longer pink on the outside (3 or 4 minutes), add the broccoli to the skillet. Cook 5 minutes more, stirring often. Remove from the heat when the chicken is done.

5 When the potatoes finish baking, cut each potato in half horizontally. Be careful — they're hot!

6 Scoop a 2-inch hollow out of each potato (save the scoopings for another snack) and sprinkle the cheese inside.

7 Fill the hollow with the chicken and broccoli. Sprinkle more cheese on top.

8 When the cheese melts, serve the taters with sour cream and salsa.

Per serving: Calories 202 (From Fat 82); Fat 9g (Saturated 4g); Cholesterol 39mg; Sodium 709mg; Carbohydrate 17g (Dietary Fiber 1.5g); Protein 15g.

Tip: These taters are delicious cold, too! Take one to work for a snack. If you prefer them warm, they reheat well in the microwave.

Vary It! Try this recipe with roasted red potatoes instead of russets (you'll have to decrease the bake time to approximately 30 minutes).

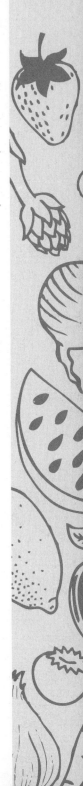

Turkey Nachos

Prep time: 5 min • **Cook time:** 15 min • **Yield:** 6–8 servings

Ingredients	*Directions*
½ pound ground turkey	**1** Coat a medium skillet with no-stick cooking spray. Combine the turkey, onion, and peppers in the skillet. Cook over medium heat, stirring often, until the turkey is browned (about 7 minutes).
½ cup chopped onion	
½ cup chopped red pepper	
½ cup chopped green or jalapeño pepper	
2 tablespoons taco seasoning mix	**2** Stir in the taco seasoning and water and simmer 5 to 7 minutes, stirring occasionally, until the water has cooked down.
⅓ cup water	
5 ounces blue corn chips	**3** Pile the corn chips on a large plate. Top with the turkey and pepper mix. Sprinkle with the cheese.
4 ounces shredded Mexican cheese blend	
1 tomato, diced	**4** Microwave the nachos until the cheese is melted. Top with tomato and avocado and serve warm with sour cream and salsa (if desired).
½ avocado, diced	
Sour cream or fresh salsa (optional)	

Per serving: Calories 244 (From Fat 113); Fat 12g (Saturated 5g); Cholesterol 45mg; Sodium 343mg; Carbohydrate 19g (Dietary Fiber 2.5g); Protein 14g.

Toasted Nori Chips with Salmon

Prep time: 15 min • **Cook time:** 10–15 min • **Yield:** 4–6 servings (about 48 crisps)

Ingredients	Directions
3 ounce wild-caught salmon filet	*1* Preheat the oven to 250 degrees. Cut the salmon into very thin strips (¹⁄₁₆ inch to ⅛ inch thick). Use a fork to hold the salmon so you don't cut your fingers!
2 tablespoons powdered wasabi horseradish	*2* In a small bowl, whisk the wasabi and water together until dissolved. Wasabi settles, so you'll have to re-whisk often during preparation.
¼ cup water	
8 sheets nori (sushi seaweed wrap)	*3* Fold one sheet of nori in half. Unfold it and brush half the sheet with wasabi water. Add slivers of salmon, sprinkle with sea salt, and fold closed.
Sea salt	
	4 Brush the top of the closed sheet with wasabi water.
	5 Cut the sheet into six strips and transfer them to a baking sheet.
	6 Repeat Steps 3 through 5 until the baking sheet is filled. Don't allow the nori strips to touch one another on the sheet.
	7 Bake for 10 to 15 minutes, until the nori is dark and brittle.
	8 Remove the strips from the oven and transfer them to a cooling rack. Serve at room temperature after the crisps cool. To store, refrigerate them in an airtight container.

Per serving: Calories 25 (From Fat 8); Fat 1g (Saturated 0.5g); Cholesterol 2.5mg; Sodium 150mg; Carbohydrate 1.5g (Dietary Fiber 1g); Protein 4g.

Vary It! If the salmon inside the crisps is too undercooked for your taste, brown it in a skillet with a dot of olive oil before inserting it into the wrap.

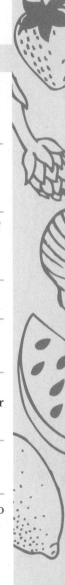

Veggie Burger Patties

Prep time: 10 min • **Cook time:** 10 min • **Yield:** 2 servings

Ingredients	Directions
No-stick canola spray	**1** Preheat the oven to 475 degrees. Grease a small cookie sheet with no-stick canola spray.
½ cup cooked garbanzo beans	
1 teaspoon tomato paste	**2** In a blender, mix the garbanzo beans, tomato paste, Worcestershire, garlic powder, salt, and pepper.
½ teaspoon Worcestershire sauce	
1 pinch garlic powder	**3** Add the bulgur, onion, parsley, mushrooms, and chives. Mix again, only until just blended.
1 pinch salt	
1 pinch ground black pepper	**4** Flatten the bean mix into two 3-to-4-inch patties and bake them on the cookie sheet for about 5 minutes. Flip each patty and bake another 5 minutes until slightly crisp.
¾ cup cooked bulgur	
1 tablespoon minced red onion	
1 teaspoon minced fresh parsley	
1 tablespoon chopped mushrooms of choice	
1 tablespoon minced chives	

Per serving: Calories 129 (From Fat 65); Fat 7g (Saturated 0.5g); Cholesterol 0mg; Sodium 621mg; Carbohydrate 15g (Dietary Fiber 3.5g); Protein 2.5g.

Tip: This patty recipe goes well with many different condiments, like horseradish, steak sauce, mustard, or Tabasco sauce.

Vary It! Worcestershire sauce contains anchovies, so for a vegan variation, substitute soy sauce.

Baby Shrimp Salad with Dill Dressing

Prep time: 6 min • **Cook time:** 7 min • **Yield:** 4 servings

Ingredients	Directions
¾ cup white wine	**1** In a 2- or 3-quart saucepan, combine the wine, bay leaves, and lemon slices. Add water to the pan until it's half full. Bring to a boil over high heat.
2 bay leaves	
1 fresh lemon, sliced	
1 pound baby shrimp, peeled and deveined	**2** Add the shrimp and boil 1 to 2 minutes, until the shrimp are pink.
Dill Dressing (see the following recipe)	**3** Drain the shrimp in a strainer and cool them under cold water. Remove the bay leaves and lemon pieces.
Salt and ground black pepper to taste	**4** Place the shrimp in a clean bowl and add the dressing. Salt and pepper to taste. Toss well. Refrigerate and serve chilled.

Dill Dressing

3 tablespoons olive oil	**1** In a medium bowl, whisk together all the ingredients. Optional: Shake vigorously in a shaker cup instead of whisking in a bowl.
3 tablespoons red wine vinegar	
1 tablespoon chopped fresh basil	
2 tablespoons chopped fresh dill	
½ medium onion, chopped	
1 teaspoon Dijon mustard	

Per serving: Calories 258 (From Fat 107); Fat 12g (Saturated 2g); Cholesterol 41mg; Sodium 833mg; Carbohydrate 17g (Dietary Fiber 2g); Protein 15g.

Tip: Serve on a bed of fresh lettuce or on multigrain crackers.

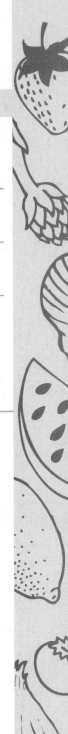

Guacamole

Prep time: 10 min • **Yield:** 2 servings (1 cup each)

Ingredients	*Directions*
2 avocados, diced	*1* In a medium bowl, mash the avocado with the back of a fork or a potato masher. Mix in the remaining ingredients, except the chips or pita. Salt and pepper to taste. Serve with corn chips or pita wedges.
½ cup fresh salsa	
1 tablespoon sour cream or plain Greek yogurt	
¼ cup chopped fresh cilantro	
2 tablespoons fresh lime juice	
1 tablespoon taco seasoning	
1 pinch garlic powder	
½ cup shredded jack or pepper jack cheese	
5 kalamata or black olives, pitted and chopped (optional)	
Salt and ground black pepper to taste	
Corn chips or pita wedges for serving	

Per serving: Calories 199 (From Fat 123); Fat 14g (Saturated 6g); Cholesterol 33mg; Sodium 794mg; Carbohydrate 11g (Dietary Fiber 2.5g); Protein 10g.

Tip: This guacamole makes a great topping for a baked potato.

Spinach Quiche Cups

Prep time: 10 min • **Cook time:** 25 min • **Yield:** 8 servings

Ingredients	Directions
No-stick spray	**1** Preheat the oven to 350 degrees. Grease 8 muffin cups with no-stick spray.
8 ounces frozen spinach	
2 eggs	**2** Cook the spinach in the microwave according to the package directions. Squeeze well to drain excess water.
¾ cup shredded cheese of choice	
¼ cup diced green bell pepper	**3** In a medium bowl, beat the eggs thoroughly. Add the spinach, cheese, peppers, and mushrooms. Salt and pepper to taste. Mix well and divide evenly into mixing cups.
1 teaspoon minced jalapeño pepper (optional)	
¼ cup diced mushrooms	
Salt and ground black pepper to taste	**4** Bake for 20 minutes, until a toothpick inserted into the center comes out clean.

Per serving: Calories 78 (From Fat 45); Fat 5g (Saturated 2.5g); Cholesterol 57mg; Sodium 288mg; Carbohydrate 1.5g (Dietary Fiber 0.5g); Protein 5g.

Vary It! For more protein, add ¼ cup cooked crumbled sausage to Step 3.

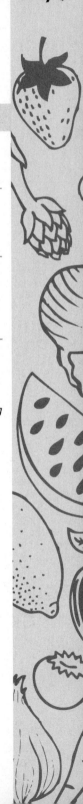

Cheesesteak Slabs

Prep time: 10 min • **Cook time:** 10 min • **Yield:** 4 servings

Ingredients	Directions
4 to 6 ounces cooked steak	*1* Chip or shave the steak with a knife and fork or with a vegetable peeler and fork.
1 tablespoon butter	
¼ cup sliced green bell pepper	*2* In a medium skillet, heat the butter over medium-high heat until it's melted. Sauté the pepper, onion, and mushrooms until the peppers are tender, about 5 minutes, stirring often. Salt and pepper to taste.
2 tablespoons sliced onion	
½ cup sliced mushrooms of choice	
Salt and ground black pepper to taste	*3* Add the steak shavings to the vegetables and sauté 1 minute more, stirring constantly. Remove from heat.
4 slices Melba toast	*4* Coat each slice of Melba toast with mustard and cover with the steak mix. Top with half a slice of provolone cheese.
1 tablespoon spicy mustard	
2 thin slices provolone cheese	
	5 Heat the slabs in a toaster oven or an oven heated to 300 degrees, until the cheese is melted. Serve hot.

Per serving: Calories 204 (From Fat 123); Fat 14g (Saturated 7g); Cholesterol 49mg; Sodium 499mg; Carbohydrate 6g (Dietary Fiber 1g); Protein 14g.

Vary It! This recipe is designed for leftover steak, but it's also delicious with thin slices of leftover chicken, pork, or turkey. For something different, substitute banana pepper for green pepper.

Chapter 17

Sin-Free Desserts

In This Chapter

▶ Changing your dessert habits to healthier fare

▶ Upgrading your definition of dessert

Dessert. The word inspires excitement in some and dread in others. For some people, finishing every meal by indulging in a sweet decadence has become a lifelong habit. Others eat desserts infrequently but go overboard whenever sugary delights are present. The holiday season can be a nightmare (or a dream come true) for dessert-o-holics because December tends to bring cookies, candies, and sweet goodies around every corner.

You're taking steps to reduce or eliminate sugar from your diet, but that doesn't mean that you have to swear off desserts forever. You can make smart choices to have your dessert and eat it too. This chapter provides some tips to lower the sugar content of the desserts you enjoy. I also offer some ideas to help shift your perception of what dessert can be, so that you can pick healthier alternatives when you decide to indulge in some extra calories.

All the dessert recipes in this chapter are free of processed sugars and artificial sweeteners, but some contain more natural sugar than other recipes in this book. The sugar content in the nutritional analysis section reflects the use of fruit, fruit juice, or honey in these recipes.

Whenever possible, you should try to use organic ingredients, hormone-free dairy, and pasture-fed eggs in these recipes.

Practicing Sugar-Free Satisfaction

Many sugar cravings stem purely from habit — the more sugar you eat, the more you want. When you eat dessert every day, you continue to want dessert every day.

Don't make after-dinner sweets an everyday habit. When you feel like having something sweet after a meal, drink some flavored mineral water or herbal tea instead, or pick a low-sugar alternative from the following list. Reserve the heavy-sugar desserts for very special occasions, if at all. After you start weaning yourself off your daily sugar overload, you'll probably find that those sickly sweet monstrosities aren't very appealing anymore.

Having something sweet after a meal doesn't mean that you have to cram a thousand calories of Chocolate Mountain Thunder on top of your dinner! You love dessert as much as the next person (okay, maybe a lot more), but you have plenty of sensible ways to indulge your sweet tooth without assaulting your pancreas.

The first two bites of anything are the most satisfying. You can teach yourself to be content with just a few small bites of something that is sweet and pleasurable but that doesn't have added sugar. Next time you feel the drive to experience something sweet, try one of these alternatives:

- A few bites of chilled mango
- One piece of sugar-free chocolate topped with pistachio and sea salt
- Three bite-sized pieces of banana topped with almond butter
- Two strawberries

The allure of dessert isn't really about what you're specifically eating; it's about the experience of having something sweet. When you focus on the sensations of the dessert experience (be sure to read Chapter 8 on mindful eating), you get a lot more satisfaction out of the experience, and you need a lot less sugar to feel satisfied. Two bites of sensory overload will be all you can handle!

Another strategy I've developed that works well for many people is to allow one junk food item per day (once per day for now — after you break your sugar addiction, you can move toward once per week). Your junk food choice can be a traditional dessert or another low-nutrition item like potato chips or French fries. The once-per-day system works well because it coaxes you out of the dessert mentality — the Pavlovian habit of always wanting something sweet at the end of your meal. Focusing on junk food breaks the timing-dependent habit of dessert and encourages planning and decision-making because you only get one indulgence per day.

While you're learning to break the habit of eating something sweet after every meal, be sure to use the flowchart in Chapter 9 that walks you through exactly what to do when a sugar craving strikes.

Applesauce Cookies

Prep time: 15 min • **Cook time:** 8–10 min • **Yield:** 4 dozen cookies

Ingredients	*Directions*
2 cups unbleached white flour	*1* Preheat the oven to 350 degrees. Line a cookie sheet with parchment paper. (Prepare two cookie sheets if you're able to bake two trays at once.)
½ teaspoon baking powder	
1 teaspoon cinnamon	
2 tablespoons unsweetened coconut flakes	*2* In a mixing bowl, mix together the flour, baking powder, cinnamon, coconut, and nutmeg.
½ teaspoon nutmeg	
2 eggs	*3* Add the eggs, vegetable oil, applesauce, and apple juice concentrate. Beat well.
2 tablespoons vegetable oil	
1 cup unsweetened applesauce	*4* Stir in the granola.
2 tablespoons unsweetened apple juice concentrate	*5* Drop the batter by teaspoons onto the cookie sheet.
2 cups unsweetened granola	*6* Bake at 350 degrees for 8 to 10 minutes, until the cookie bottoms are brown and the centers are firm.
	7 Remove the cookie sheets from the oven and allow cookies to rest on the sheet for 1 minute. Transfer the cookies to wire racks to cool.

Per serving: Calories 53 (From Fat 21); Fat 2.5g (Saturated 0.5g); Cholesterol 8mg; Sodium 11mg; Carbohydrate 7g (Dietary Fiber 0.5g); Protein 1.5g.

Vary It! Add ¼ cup chopped figs to Step 4.

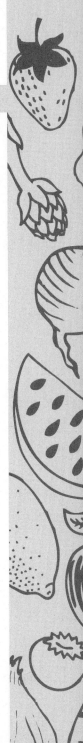

Vegan Peanut Butter Cookies

Prep time: 15 min • **Cook time:** 15 min • **Yield:** 4 dozen cookies

Ingredients	Directions
2½ cups rolled oats	**1** Preheat the oven to 350 degrees. Line a cookie sheet with parchment paper. (Prepare two cookie sheets if you're able to bake two trays at once.)
¼ cup all-purpose flour	
⅛ teaspoon cinnamon	
2 mashed bananas	**2** In large mixing bowl, stir together the oats, flour, and cinnamon.
⅓ cup creamy peanut butter	
2 tablespoons unsweetened soy milk	**3** In a separate bowl, combine the mashed bananas, peanut butter, soy milk, oil, maple syrup, and vanilla extract. Mix well.
¼ cup vegetable oil	
2 tablespoons pure maple syrup	**4** Combine the banana mixture and the oat mixture and mix well.
1 teaspoon pure vanilla extract	**5** Drop the batter by teaspoons onto the cookie sheet.
	6 Bake at 350 degrees for approximately 15 minutes, until firm. Be careful not to let the edges burn.
	7 Remove the cookies from the oven and transfer them to wire racks to cool.

Per serving: Calories 49 (From Fat 21); Fat 2.5g (Saturated 0.5g); Cholesterol 0mg; Sodium 17mg; Carbohydrate 6g (Dietary Fiber 0.5g); Protein 1g.

Chocolate Oatmeal Cookies

Prep time: 10 min • **Cook time:** 12–15 min • **Yield:** 4 dozen cookies

Ingredients	Directions
1 cup whole-wheat flour	**1** Preheat the oven to 375 degrees. Line a cookie sheet with parchment paper. (Prepare two cookie sheets if you're able to bake two trays at once.)
1 cup rolled oats	
1 cup unsweetened applesauce	**2** In a large mixing bowl, combine all ingredients and mix well.
½ cup raisins	
½ cup dark chocolate chips or chopped dark chocolate chunks	**3** Drop the batter by teaspoons onto the cookie sheet.
¼ cup chopped macadamia nuts	**4** Bake for 12 to 15 minutes, until brown.
2 eggs	**5** Remove the cookies from the oven and transfer them to wire racks to cool.
1 teaspoon ground cinnamon	
1 teaspoon baking powder	
½ teaspoon baking soda	
¼ teaspoon nutmeg	
¼ teaspoon allspice	
⅓ cup vegetable oil	
¼ cup water	
1 teaspoon pure vanilla extract	

Per serving: *Calories 52 (From Fat 25); Fat 3g (Saturated 0.5g); Cholesterol 8mg; Sodium 18mg; Carbohydrate 6g (Dietary Fiber 0.5g); Protein 1g.*

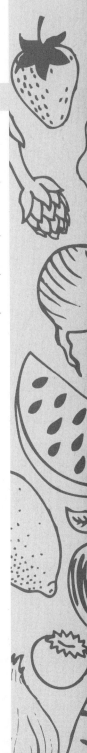

Pineapple Carrot Cookies

Prep time: 10 min • **Cook time:** 10–12 min • **Yield:** 4 dozen cookies

Ingredients	Directions
2 cups whole-wheat flour	**1** Preheat the oven to 350 degrees. Line a cookie sheet with parchment paper. (Prepare two cookie sheets if you're able to bake two trays at once.)
1½ teaspoons baking soda	
½ teaspoon nutmeg	
¾ teaspoon ginger	**2** In a large bowl, mix together the flour, baking soda, nutmeg, ginger, cinnamon, and oats. Mix in the carrots, pineapple, and raisins.
1 teaspoon cinnamon	
¾ cup rolled oats	
1 cup grated carrots	**3** In a separate large mixing bowl, combine the butter, egg white, vanilla extract, and apple and pineapple juice concentrates. Beat well.
¾ cup crushed pineapple, drained	
¾ cup raisins	**4** Add the oat and carrot mixture to the butter mixture, and beat until well blended.
3 tablespoons butter, softened	
1 egg white	**5** Drop the batter by teaspoons onto the cookie sheet.
½ teaspoon pure vanilla extract	
¼ cup unsweetened apple juice concentrate	**6** Bake for 10 to 12 minutes, until browned.
½ cup unsweetened pineapple juice concentrate	

Per serving: Calories 44 (From Fat 8); Fat 1g (Saturated 0.5g); Cholesterol 2mg; Sodium 23mg; Carbohydrate 2g (Dietary Fiber 1g); Protein 1g.

Vary It! For moister cookies, add ¼ cup vegetable oil to Step 3.

Sugar-Free Brownies

Prep time: 10 min • **Cook time:** 30 min • **Yield:** 12 servings

Ingredients	Directions
1 tablespoon butter (to grease pan)	**1** Preheat the oven to 350 degrees. Grease the inside of a 9-x-13-inch baking pan with butter.
1 cup whole-wheat flour	
¼ cup cocoa	**2** In a large mixing bowl, sift together the flour, cocoa, and baking powder.
½ teaspoon baking powder	
⅔ cup unsweetened apple juice concentrate	**3** Add the apple juice concentrate, oil, egg, walnuts, and banana. Mix well.
¼ cup canola or vegetable oil	
1 egg white	**4** Spread the batter into the prepared pan. Bake at 350 degrees for 30 minutes.
¼ cup chopped walnuts	
1 mashed banana	**5** Remove the brownies from the oven and allow them to cool for a few minutes in the pan before cutting. Serve warm.

Per serving: Calories 139 (From Fat 68); Fat 8g (Saturated 1.5g); Cholesterol 2.5mg; Sodium 18mg; Carbohydrate 17g (Dietary Fiber 2g); Protein 2.5g.

Insulin-friendly baking tips

To turn high-glycemic or high-sugar desserts into low-sugar, insulin-friendly treats, try these healthier substitutions:

- ✔ Add whey protein or nuts for extra protein and better blood sugar control.

- ✔ Look for ways to add grated carrots, apples, or pumpkin in recipes to add more fiber and moisture, while cutting back on the sugar.

- ✔ Substitute half the flour called for in a recipe with whole-grain flour like oat flour, brown rice flour, or spelt.

- ✔ To cut back on calories, replace oil with unsweetened applesauce (using the same measurement), or use only ¾ the amount of oil called for in the recipe.

- ✔ Try decreasing the amount of sugar used in a recipe by 25 to 50 percent of what's called for.

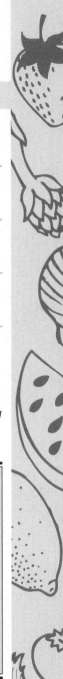

Zucchini Muffins

Prep time: 10 min • **Cook time:** 20 min • **Yield:** 18 muffins

Ingredients	Directions
1½ cups grated zucchini, patted dry	**1** Preheat the oven to 325 degrees.
1½ cups rolled oats	**2** In a large mixing bowl, combine the zucchini, oats, flour, baking soda, cream of tartar, nutmeg, and cinnamon.
1½ cups whole-wheat flour	
2 teaspoons baking soda	
2 teaspoons cream of tartar	**3** In a separate bowl, combine the honey, applesauce, pineapple, cranberries, vanilla extract, egg whites, and pineapple juice concentrate.
¼ teaspoon nutmeg	
2 teaspoons ground cinnamon	
¼ cup honey	**4** Combine the wet mixture with the dry mixture, stirring only until combined — don't whip.
¾ cup unsweetened applesauce	
8 ounces crushed pineapple, drained	**5** Apportion 18 muffins into muffin pans lined with muffin papers.
¼ cup chopped dried cranberries	**6** In a small bowl, mix the pecans and flax meal. Top each muffin with ½ teaspoon of the nut-and-flax mix.
1 teaspoon pure vanilla extract	
2 egg whites	**7** Bake for 20 minutes, until a toothpick inserted into the center of a muffin comes out clean.
¼ cup unsweetened pineapple juice concentrate	
¼ cup pecans, chopped	
2 tablespoons flax meal	

Per serving: Calories 123 (From Fat 18); Fat 2g (Saturated 0g); Cholesterol 0mg; Sodium 148mg; Carbohydrate 25g (Dietary Fiber 2g); Protein 3g.

Vary It! Substitute raisins for the chopped cranberries.

Banana Nut Bread

Prep time: 15 min • **Cook time:** 55 min • **Yield:** 16 slices

Ingredients	Directions
1 teaspoon butter (to grease pan)	*1* Preheat the oven to 325 degrees. Grease the inside of a 9-x-5-inch loaf pan with butter.
2 cups all-purpose flour	
1 scoop whey protein powder (vanilla or unflavored)	*2* In a mixing bowl, mix together the flour, whey protein, baking soda, baking powder, cinnamon, and nutmeg.
1 teaspoon baking soda	
2 teaspoons baking powder	
½ teaspoon ground cinnamon	*3* Add the banana, oil, eggs, vanilla extract, and water. Beat well until creamy.
½ teaspoon nutmeg	
¾ cup mashed bananas	*4* Stir in the walnuts.
⅓ cup vegetable oil	
2 eggs	*5* Pour the batter into the prepared loaf pan. Spread the batter evenly.
1 teaspoon pure vanilla extract	
½ cup water	*6* Bake at 325 degrees for approximately 55 minutes, until a knife inserted into the center comes out clean.
1 cup chopped walnuts	
	7 Remove the loaf from the pan and cool completely on a wire rack before serving.

Per serving: Calories 167 (From Fat 95); Fat 11g (Saturated 1.5g); Cholesterol 24mg; Sodium 294mg; Carbohydrate 15g (Dietary Fiber 1g); Protein 4g.

Vary It! Add ¼ cup of raisins to Step 4.

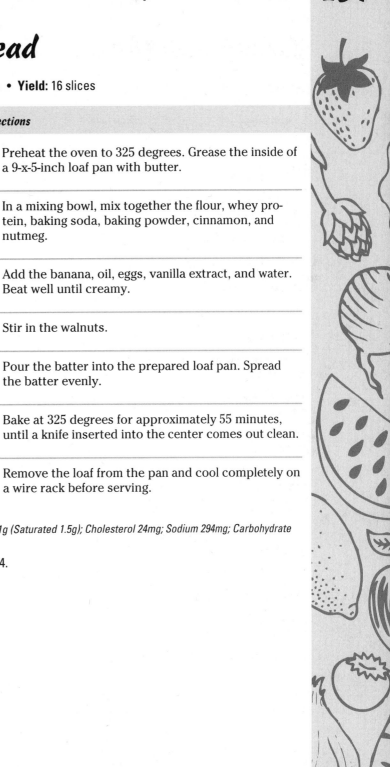

Frozen Strawberry Banana Treat

Prep time: 5 min • **Yield:** 1 serving

Ingredients	*Directions*
¼ **cup skim milk**	**1** Place the milk, banana, strawberries, whey protein, and ice cubes in a food processor and blend until smooth and whipped.
½ **frozen banana**	
3 **large strawberries, cored**	
1 **scoop whey protein powder (vanilla or unflavored)**	**2** Core the apple and chop it into ½-inch cubes. Place in serving bowl.
2 **ice cubes**	
½ **apple, any variety**	**3** Using a rubber spatula, scrape the frozen treat onto the apple pieces and enjoy.

Per serving: Calories 275 (From Fat 20); Fat 2g (Saturated 1g); Cholesterol 51mg; Sodium 68mg; Carbohydrate 46g (Dietary Fiber 6g); Protein 22g.

Tip: Sprinkle a little fresh chopped mint on top.

Black Forest Parfait

Prep time: 10 min • **Cook time:** 10 min • **Yield:** 4 servings

Ingredients	Directions
4 ounces dark chocolate (70% cacao), flaked and divided	**1** Chill four parfait glasses in the freezer. Measure 2 tablespoons of the chocolate flakes and set aside.
8 ounces frozen no-sugar-added pitted cherries	**2** In a medium saucepan, heat the cherries over medium heat. As the cherries start to thaw, simmer until the juice is released, taking care not to let them burn. Remove them from the heat when they are warm and soft.
¼ teaspoon pure vanilla extract	
¼ cup roasted unsalted cashew pieces	
1 teaspoon stevia powder	**3** To the cherries, stir in the vanilla extract, cashew pieces, and the remaining chocolate flakes. Allow the mixture to cool slightly but not harden, and then stir in the stevia powder to taste.
4 cups vanilla Greek yogurt	
	4 Coat each parfait cup with the chocolate cherry mix, and then add alternating layers of yogurt and sauce.
	5 Top each parfait with the remaining chocolate flakes and serve cold.

Per serving: Calories 486 (From Fat 167); Fat 19g (Saturated 8g); Cholesterol 1mg; Sodium 122mg; Carbohydrate 52g (Dietary Fiber 4g); Protein 28g.

Vary It! This parfait is also delicious with blackberries or raspberries instead of cherries. Try it with hazelnuts instead of cashews.

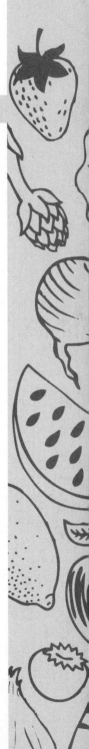

Champagne Vanilla Berry Pudding

Prep time: 10 min • **Cook time:** 15 min • **Yield:** 4 servings

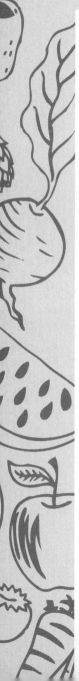

Ingredients	Directions
3 tablespoons cornstarch	*1* In a large bowl, prepare an ice bath to fit a medium bowl that will sit inside it. Set aside.
½ teaspoon stevia powder	
2 eggs	*2* In a medium mixing bowl, whisk together the cornstarch and stevia. Add the eggs and mix well.
2 cups skim milk	
1 teaspoon pure vanilla extract	*3* In a medium saucepan, bring the milk to a boil over medium-high heat, stirring constantly. Don't allow the milk to burn — if any burned milk collects at the bottom of the saucepan, start this step over.
1 tablespoon butter	
3 tablespoons champagne or prosecco	*4* Stir a few tablespoons of the hot milk into the egg mixture to gently warm the eggs without scrambling them. Then slowly pour in the remaining milk, stirring as you pour, and mix well.
Berry Sauce (see the following recipe)	
Whipped cream (optional)	*5* Pour the milk mix back into the saucepan and whisk over medium-high heat for approximately 2 minutes, until thickened. Remove from heat.
	6 With a rubber spatula, scrape the thickened pudding into a medium bowl and whisk in the vanilla extract, butter, and champagne. Add additional stevia powder to taste if needed.
	7 Set the pudding bowl into the ice bath until chilled, stirring occasionally. Remove it from the ice and set it in the refrigerator.
	8 When the pudding and Berry Sauce are both chilled, coat parfait glasses (or other glassware) with the berry sauce and scoop in alternating layers of pudding and berry sauce. Top with a dollop of whipped cream (if desired). Serve chilled.

Berry Sauce

12 ounces frozen blueberries

12 ounces frozen strawberries or raspberries

1–2 tablespoons cornstarch

2 tablespoons chopped pecans

1 In two small separate saucepans, add the berries, one fruit in each. Add a splash of water into each pan.

2 Heat the berries over medium-high heat until boiling (approximately 5 minutes). They should become saucy, and the berries may burst. Mash large pieces of the berries with a fork to smooth out the sauce.

3 Remove the berries from the heat and transfer them into two separate bowls. Stir in the cornstarch to thicken.

4 Allow the berries to cool to room temperature and then stir in the pecans. Refrigerate until ready to use.

Per serving: Calories 306 (From Fat 80); Fat 9g (Saturated 3g); Cholesterol 102mg; Sodium 126mg; Carbohydrate 47g (Dietary Fiber 4g); Protein 9g.

Tip: You can double or triple this recipe using the same ratios.

Vary It! You can try using fresh berries instead of frozen, but be careful not to burn them. You may need to add a little extra water when cooking fresh berries.

Vary It! You can keep the berry sauces separate to make different parfait layers or combine both berries in one saucepan when you make the sauce. It's also delicious with some dark chocolate shavings on top!

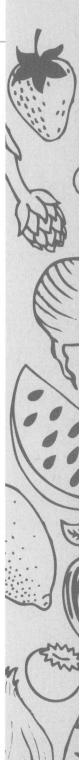

Part V
The Part of Tens

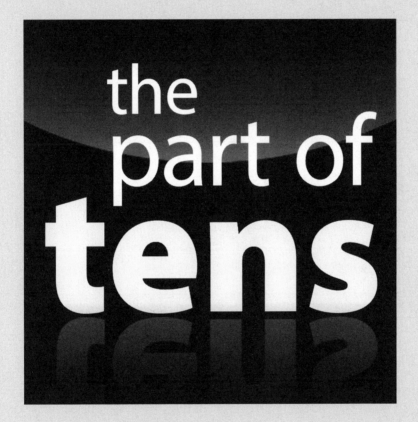

 Boost your metabolism with ten sugar-busting workout circuits at www.dummies. com/extras/beatingsugaraddiction.

In this part . . .

- ✔ Figure out which sugar-laden and just plain unhealthy foods to leave at the store when food shopping.

- ✔ Outwit your sugar cravings with smart habits like drinking more water and choosing healthy snacks.

Chapter 18

Ten Surprising Foods to Leave at the Grocery Store

In This Chapter

▶ Staying away from diet sodas, frozen entrees, and other unhealthy foods

▶ Avoiding genetically modified products

▶ Choosing truly healthy alternatives to supposedly healthy foods

*U*nless you grow your own vegetables and raise your own livestock, the grocery store is where you make primary food decisions for you and your family. Though most people recognize the junk-food quality of obvious high-sugar foods like candy and ice cream, many unhealthy items are available in the stores that you may erroneously think of as healthier alternatives. This chapter explains ten of these foods that, on the surface, may appear to be healthy choices, but in reality are not. When you come across these foods in the grocery store, keep walking!

If you're interested in making a complete dietary overhaul to all-natural foods, check out *Eating Clean For Dummies,* by Dr. Jonathan Wright and Linda Larsen (Wiley).

Diet Soda

Diet sodas are sugar-free and calorie-free, so they must be a healthier alternative to sugared soda pop, right? Wrong.

Diet drinks are artificially sweetened with aspartame (NutraSweet), a chemical that causes brain damage and can increase appetite. The type of caramel coloring used in many diet sodas is a carcinogen. The phosphoric acid in sodas leeches calcium out of your bones, contributing to osteoporosis. Stay away from sodas of all types, both sugared and zero-calorie!

If you like the fizz of soda, drink mineral water instead. You can flavor it with fresh lemon or lime.

To gradually wean yourself off of sweetened drinks, try adding stevia powder instead of sugar or chemical sweeteners to your beverages. *Stevia* is a natural, plant-based sweetener that has virtually no calories and doesn't carry the health risks that artificial sweeteners do. Over time you can gradually decrease the amount of stevia powder that you put in your water, coffee, or tea, until you don't feel like you need any added flavoring any more.

Frozen Entrees

"Healthy" frozen meals became popular in the 1980s, as food manufacturers tried to capitalize on consumers' desire for healthier alternatives to TV dinners. Because today's brands of health-conscious entrees are low in fat and calories, many dieters believe that they're making a smart decision by eating these handy products. A quick look at the ingredients list shows that this isn't the case.

For example, I selected a glazed chicken entree from the most popular line of "healthy" frozen foods at the grocery store. It's a low-calorie dinner, so I guess you could call it lean, but it sure isn't healthy. Here are some of the issues I have with the ingredients in this frozen entree:

- ✔ The chicken tenderloins undoubtedly come from feedlot meat, loaded with antibiotics, hormones, and chemicals (see Chapter 6).
- ✔ The chicken is coated with high-fructose corn syrup, several preservatives, salt, and artificial caramel color.
- ✔ The rice accompanying the chicken is blanched, enriched rice, meaning that all the nutrients have been stripped away, leaving just the carbohydrate shell. It also contains partially hydrogenated oil (trans fats), sugar, maltodextrin (more sugar), and caramel coloring.
- ✔ The vegetables are green beans with "natural flavors" (which can be anything, often a code for monosodium glutamate, or MSG) and wheat berries (probably from genetically modified wheat).

To top it all off, you're supposed to microwave the whole entree in the accompanying plastic tray. When plastics are heated, toxic chemicals leak out. Although the amount of chemicals released from microwave-safe plastics is reported to be a tiny, safe amount, these chemicals are proven carcinogens and endocrine disruptors, so I suggest you don't expose yourself or your family to them if you don't have to. Heat your food in glass containers instead.

Frozen dinners don't really save much time — it doesn't take long to chop up some organic chicken and vegetables and make a stir-fry with fresh ingredients that you control. Taking a few minutes to throw together a homemade meal like this ensures that you eat healthy ingredients and avoid dangerous chemicals.

Bacon

Bacon experienced a rise in popularity during the latest resurgence of the Atkins diet. Though a high-protein breakfast is desirable, you can find much healthier protein sources than bacon.

Conventional bacon is made from feedlot hogs and is usually loaded with nitrites and other preservatives, sugars, artificial smoke flavoring, chemical coloring, and MSG. Ounce for ounce, bacon is mostly fat and chemicals.

If you really love bacon, find a local farmer who can sell you bacon that's made without harmful chemicals from animals that are raised on good food without hormones.

Canned Soups

A piping hot bowl of chicken soup or chili sounds like a healthy meal. Even though meat and vegetables are the primary ingredients, canned soup typically contains feedlot meat, too much salt, genetically modified ingredients, high-fructose corn syrup, MSG, and preservatives.

Many companies still use cans with *bisphenol-a* (BPA) in the lining. BPA is a chemical that acts as an artificial estrogen and has been linked to several negative health consequences.

If you don't want to make your own soup, look for brands that are made from organic ingredients, without chemical additives, and that are canned in BPA-free containers.

Genetically Modified Foods

In the 1990s, food manufacturers began using plants that had gone through a process of genetic engineering — inserting genes from other plants, animals, or bacteria to alter the crop's genome. Foods that have been genetically modified — often referred to as *GM foods* or *GMOs* (genetically modified organisms) — have caused concern among some members of the scientific community for possible human and environmental health risks, such as infertility, organ damage, and immune system problems.

No one knows for certain what harm these products will end up causing to people's bodies and the environment. My guess is that certain modifications are probably harmless, but some of them are certainly not. Unfortunately, only time will tell. In the meantime, I advise you to stay away from genetically engineered food products whenever possible. By law, food labeled "100 percent organic" can't contain genetically modified ingredients, so look for that label when shopping. Better yet, find a local farmer who raises nonmodified crops.

In 1988, more than 60 countries voted unanimously against the use of GMOs in food production and agriculture because the scientific consensus was that unacceptable risks were involved: threats to human health, a negative and irreversible environmental impact, and incompatibility with sustainable agriculture practices. Twenty-five years later, the United States still doesn't require genetically modified foods to be labeled as such. If you think that Americans should have a right to know what's in their food, contact your congressperson!

PLU (price lookup code) stickers on produce tell you whether the food was conventionally grown, genetically modified, or organically grown. The PLU code for conventional produce is four numbers, while genetically modified produce has five numbers, starting with the number 8. Organically grown produce has five numbers, starting with the number 9.

Microwave Popcorn

You may consider popcorn to be a low-calorie, high-fiber snack, but microwave popcorn isn't a healthy choice. When microwaved, popcorn bags leak *perfluorooctanoic acid* (PFOA) and other plastic residues into your food. PFOA has been linked to infertility, thyroid disease, and a host of other endocrine disorders.

Aside from the packaging, commercial microwave popcorn typically contains harmful trans fats, preservatives, artificial colors, sugar, chemical sweeteners, and other "flavor enhancers" like MSG. Read the ingredients once and you'll never touch a bag again.

To avoid dangerous chemicals, pop your own non-GMO corn at home with an air popper. If you like, add organic butter and sea salt.

Fruit Juice and Juice Drinks

Even though fruit juice is loaded with vitamins and antioxidants, even 100 percent juice contains too much sugar to be a good choice for those who are trying to limit their sugar intake. Excess fructose (fruit sugar) causes body fat accumulation, increased appetite, liver disease, and elevated cholesterol and triglycerides. Consult Chapter 3 for more information about fructose.

Juice drinks, such as juice cocktails or juice boxes for kids, are often only 10 percent fruit juice, with the rest of the ingredients being high-fructose corn syrup and other sweeteners, artificial colors, and preservatives.

An 8-ounce glass of orange juice has approximately 25 grams of sugar. Keep this in mind when portioning your beverages. If you choose to drink fruit juice occasionally, make sure you drink 100 percent juice (with no additives), and limit yourself to a 4-ounce serving.

Rice Cakes

Any all-carbohydrate snack — especially if it's made of processed, enriched grains — causes an insulin spike followed by a blood sugar crash several hours later. Rice cakes, granola bars, and other all-carb snacks aren't good choices for sugar addicts because the lack of protein keeps them on the blood-sugar roller coaster and stimulates cravings.

Half a rice cake (whole grain, not enriched) topped with almond butter or organic cheese adds fat and protein to mitigate the insulin response and keep your blood sugar levels more stable.

Protein Bars

Most of the protein bars found on the shelves of grocery stores and health food stores are laden with sugars, syrups, preservatives, and *fractionated oils* (oils that are processed to become more saturated than they are naturally) — they're basically candy bars with added protein.

Not all protein snack bars are loaded with chemicals. Visit www.Beating SugarAddiction.com for current recommendations for healthy, all-natural snack bars.

Peanut Butter

Though natural peanut butter is a good source of healthy fats and protein, industrial peanut butter — commercial brands like Skippy and Jif — is made with hydrogenated oils (trans fats) to keep the oil from separating to the top of the jar. Industrial brands also add sugar and sometimes other additives like preservatives and flavorings.

Stick with organic, natural peanut butter. The ingredients should have no more than two items: peanuts and (maybe) salt. Refrigerate natural peanut butter after opening and stirring.

Chapter 19

Ten Ways to Outwit Your Cravings

In This Chapter
▶ Getting enough water, vegetables, exercise, and sleep
▶ Being mindful and choosing healthy alternative activities to eating

Sugar is everywhere, and resisting the urge to overindulge isn't always easy. Stress, poor nutrition, dehydration, and lack of sleep can all drive you to grab whatever sugar-laden junk food is handy. Building good habits — lifelong habits — is an essential task for staying off sugar. In this chapter, I lay out ten healthy habits and lifestyle changes that help minimize both the number and the intensity of any sugar cravings you may experience. If you make these principles part of how you live every day, soon your life as a sugar junkie will be just a distant memory!

Eat Small Amounts of Food Every Three to Four Hours

Low blood sugar can fire up cravings for high-sugar food. When blood sugar plummets, your energy drops and your brain has trouble focusing, making turning to sugar for a quick pick-me-up all too easy. Eating every three or four hours throughout the day helps keep your blood sugar levels more even and the sugar cravings at bay. You also won't be as hungry at night, so resisting late-night sweet fixes is easier.

Every time you eat, try to combine a *protein* and a *plant* (see Chapter 5).

Drink Enough Water throughout the Day

Even a small amount of dehydration can trigger the hypothalamus to activate the hunger and thirst centers. As I discuss in Chapter 5, drinking enough water — at least 64 ounces a day — is one of the easiest ways to keep sugar cravings in check. Doing so also cuts down on your desire for other, less healthy beverages.

Downing a glass of cold water is one of the first things you should do when a sugar craving strikes (check out the flowchart in Chapter 9).

Take Your Vitamins

A deficiency of one or more important vitamins or minerals can cause your brain to turn on the craving center in an attempt to take in more nutrients. A smart nutrition supplementation program ensures that you have all the vital nutrients you need to stay healthy, vibrant, and sugar-free.

Flip to Chapter 5 for an introduction to helpful nutrition supplements, and visit www.BeatingSugarAddiction.com for a list of recommended brands.

Stay Mindful

To stay on track with a sensible nutrition plan, and to avoid eating according to unconscious cues and temptations, you must remain mindful about when you eat, what you choose, and how much you consume. Before you begin eating, set out your portion so you're not eating from bags or serving dishes. Chew thoroughly, and pay careful attention to the whole experience of eating. What does your food really taste like? How does the smell affect what your mouth is doing? In between every bite, assess whether you've had enough to eat so that you're not using external cues like an empty plate to tell you when it's time to stop. Turn to Chapter 8 for a more in-depth discussion of mindful eating.

Consider learning some basic meditation techniques. They'll help you stay more centered and present throughout your whole day and help make mindful eating second nature. Check out *Meditation For Dummies* by Stephan Bodian (Wiley), which includes a CD with guided meditations.

Eat Lots of Vegetables Every Day

Most of your carbohydrates should come from vegetables. Though whole grains contain some quality nutrients, they're also higher in calories and typically have a higher glycemic load than vegetables. Fibrous vegetables like broccoli, squash, and greens are low in calories and high in nutrients and fiber, so they should make up the bulk of your carbohydrate intake.

When it comes to complete nutrition, variety is key. Refer to the fruit and vegetable color chart that I lay out in Chapter 6, and regularly try to eat a wide spectrum of vegetables and fruits of various colors.

Exercise

Regular exercise unquestionably helps you lose weight, improves your insulin sensitivity, and increases your metabolism. It can also help you look and feel great and give you something to do besides eat. If you're not comfortable at a gym, you can start doing some workouts at home or begin a modest walking program four or five days per week.

See Chapter 12 for an overview of exercise basics, and visit `www.getting fit.com` and `http://blog.gettingfit.com` for more in-depth exercise advice.

Choose a Positive Substitute Behavior When a Craving Strikes

Whenever a sugar craving strikes, making a conscious decision to do something other than eat sugar is a healthy and empowering alternative. Positive activities like exercising, learning, creating something new, connecting with friends, and helping other people give you an alternative activity to gobbling down the sweet stuff and add more love and enjoyment to a world that desperately needs it. Experiment with some of the positive substitute activities in Chapter 9 and see what floats your boat.

Avoid Boredom

Some people eat when they're bored, but mindless or reactive eating is never a good idea, especially if the convenient snacks lying around are the high-sugar or high-carb type. If your brain is craving some stimulation, give it something better to do than catatonic chewing! Keep your mind active with crossword or Sudoku puzzles, reading, creative writing, or other brain-nourishing tasks. Getting up and doing something also helps — take a walk or practice a musical instrument to replace mindless eating and to limit your consumption of extra empty calories.

If you're the type who gets bored easily, make a "go to" list of brain-stimulating activities that you enjoy. The next time boredom strikes, get your brain back in gear by picking an activity from your list.

Get Enough Sleep

Lack of sleep has been proven to contribute to increases in both body fat and appetite. Sleep deprivation also impairs problem solving, alertness, concentration, reasoning, and attention (that's why it's one of the leading causes of auto accidents and workplace injuries). When you don't sleep well, you feel tired and crave sugar to artificially generate energy. Try to get at least seven hours of solid sleep each night.

Consider a melatonin supplement before bed (*melatonin* is a hormone that helps regulate sleep patterns and looks like it may offer protection against cancer), or try a cup of valerian or chamomile tea. See Chapter 7 for more tips on optimizing quality sleep.

Don't Let Triggers Make Decisions for You

It's easy to fall into the trap of reactive behavior, including making poor food choices when you feel stressed. Much of the anxiety and stress people experience is caused purely by the stories they make up about what's happening or what they're afraid will happen. Being aware of the truth of the present situation (instead of making up stories in your head and reacting to them) is crucial to maintaining healthy eating habits and a healthy overall emotional state.

The key to overcoming stress eating (and reactive behavior in general) is to become very clear about what you really want. When you experience an emotional trigger, force yourself to do a quick reality check to determine what you really need. For example, if you feel stressed and overwhelmed, what you really want is peacefulness and personal power, not sugar. If you're unhappy with the behavior of your spouse, what you probably need is to feel reassured and reconnected with your partner — sugar can't give you that.

The simple steps to stop stress eating are as follows:

1. **Recognize when you've been triggered.**

2. **Stop and figure out what you really need.**

3. **Make a conscious — not reactive — decision.**

I invite you to really dig into Chapter 9 to get a more thorough understanding of emotional triggers and advice on how to stop the cycle of reactive behavior and stress eating. It's one of the most life-changing chapters in this book!

Appendix

Metric Conversion Guide

· ·

*N*ote: The recipes in this book weren't developed or tested using metric measurements. There may be some variation in quality when converting to metric units.

Common Abbreviations

Abbreviation(s)	What It Stands For
cm	Centimeter
C., c.	Cup
G, g	Gram
kg	Kilogram
L, l	Liter
lb.	Pound
mL, ml	Milliliter
oz.	Ounce
pt.	Pint
t., tsp.	Teaspoon
T., Tb., Tbsp.	Tablespoon

Volume

U.S. Units	Canadian Metric	Australian Metric
¼ teaspoon	1 milliliter	1 milliliter
½ teaspoon	2 milliliters	2 milliliters
1 teaspoon	5 milliliters	5 milliliters
1 tablespoon	15 milliliters	20 milliliters
¼ cup	50 milliliters	60 milliliters
⅓ cup	75 milliliters	80 milliliters
½ cup	125 milliliters	125 milliliters
⅔ cup	150 milliliters	170 milliliters
¾ cup	175 milliliters	190 milliliters
1 cup	250 milliliters	250 milliliters
1 quart	1 liter	1 liter
1½ quarts	1.5 liters	1.5 liters
2 quarts	2 liters	2 liters
2½ quarts	2.5 liters	2.5 liters
3 quarts	3 liters	3 liters
4 quarts (1 gallon)	4 liters	4 liters

Weight

U.S. Units	Canadian Metric	Australian Metric
1 ounce	30 grams	30 grams
2 ounces	55 grams	60 grams
3 ounces	85 grams	90 grams
4 ounces (¼ pound)	115 grams	125 grams
8 ounces (½ pound)	225 grams	225 grams
16 ounces (1 pound)	455 grams	500 grams (½ kilogram)

Length

Inches	Centimeters
0.5	1.5
1	2.5
2	5.0
3	7.5
4	10.0
5	12.5
6	15.0
7	17.5
8	20.5
9	23.0
10	25.5
11	28.0
12	30.5

Temperature (Degrees)

Fahrenheit	Celsius
32	0
212	100
250	120
275	140
300	150
325	160
350	180
375	190
400	200
425	220
450	230
475	240
500	260

Index

• G •